Essential Oils

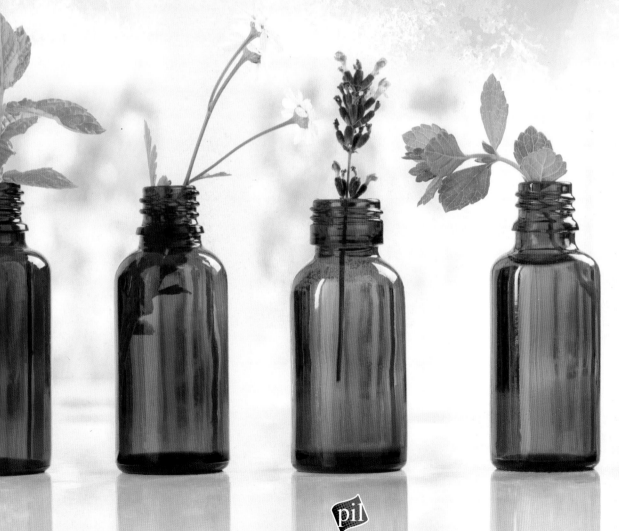

Publications International, Ltd.

Images from Alamy, Eric Bronson, Gil Nelson, Claudio Pistilli, and Shutterstock.com

Acknowledgments: Excerpt on page 15 from *The Book of Incense: Enjoying Traditional Art of Japanese Scents* by Kiyoko Morita. Published by Kodansha International, Ltd. English translation copyright © 1992 by Kodansha International Ltd. Reprinted by permission. All rights reserved.

ISBN: 978-1-64030-156-6

Manufactured in China.

8 7 6 5 4 3 2 1

Note: Neither the editors of Publications International, Ltd., nor the authors, consultants, editors, or publisher take responsibility for any possible consequence from any treatment, procedure, exercise, dietary modification, action, or application of medication or preparation by any person reading or following the information in this book. The publication of this book does not constitute the practice of medicine, and this book does not attempt to replace your physician or your pharmacist. Before undertaking any course of treatment, the authors, consultants, editors, and publisher advise the reader to check with a physician or other health care provider.

CONTENTS

INTRODUCTION

Aroma means scent, and therapy means treatment. Aromatherapy, then, is the use of the fragrant parts of aromatic plants to improve your health and general well-being. First, of course, aromatherapy offers pure enjoyment. Taking a whiff of a spice in your kitchen or a bouquet of flowers is fundamental aromatherapy.

There are many other therapeutic benefits to be gained from the use of plant essences. Inhaling the appropriate fragrance can reduce stress, lift a depression, hasten a good night's sleep, soothe your soul, or give you more energy. It can help office workers stay alert while doing repetitive mental tasks. Hospitals have experimented with using aromatherapy to help patients relax so that other healing modalities can do their job.

Massaging aromatic oils into your skin is another way to benefit from aromatherapy. That's because essential oils, the compounds responsible for a plant's fragrance, offer a multitude of healing benefits in addition to their individual scents. Many familiar plants provide us with multifaceted essential oils. Rosemary, lavender, orange, and lemon, for example, all produce essential oils that can be used therapeutically. Essential oils from these and other familiar plants are profiled and are used in therapeutic recipes throughout this book.

Essential Oils gives you the information and the tools you need to begin tapping the therapeutic properties of these amazing substances. You'll learn how to make basic healing applications, such as compresses and gargles, and you'll find specific recipes to treat a wide variety of conditions, from acne to insomnia to warts. You'll also find great ideas for diffusion blends, homemade soaps, and ways to use natural, safe essential oils as replacements for harsh cleaning chemicals.

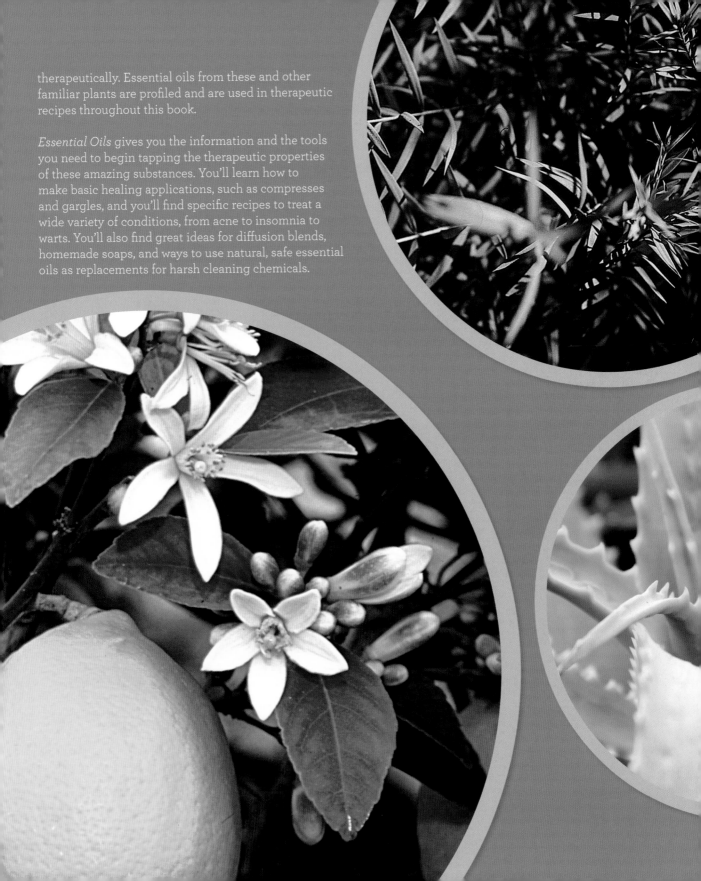

FRAGRANT ORIGINS

The earliest form of aromatherapy may have occurred through the discovery that some firewoods, such as cypress and cedar, filled the air with scent when they burned. In fact, our modern word *perfume* is derived from the Latin *per fumum*, which means "through smoke." Ancient people had probably been throwing fragrant tree needles and gums on their campfires for thousands of years by the time the first incense was developed. Incense was not the only early use of fragrance, however. Sometime between 7000 and 4000 BC, Neolithic tribes learned that animal fats, when heated, absorbed plants' aromatic and healing properties. Perhaps fragrant leaves or flowers accidentally dropped into fat as meat cooked over the fire. The information gleaned from that accident led to other discoveries: Such plants added flavor to food, helped heal wounds, and smoothed dry skin far better than nonscented fat. These fragrant fats—the forerunners of our modern massage and body lotions— scented the wearer, protected skin and hair from weather and insects, and relaxed aching muscles. They also affected people's energies and emotions.

Aromatic water, a third type of fragrant product, was actually a combination of essential oils, water, and alcohol. It was used to enhance the complexion and scent the skin and hair. It also was ingested as a medicinal tonic. It was the forerunner of our modern perfume.

As civilization became more advanced, incense, body oils, and aromatic waters were combined into blends to heal the mind, body, and spirit. Thus, throughout the world, aroma became an integral part of healing and laid the foundation for our use of aromatherapy today.

THE FRAGRANCE TRADE

In ancient times, commonly used essential oils such as frankincense, eucalyptus, ginger, and patchouli came from the furthest reaches of the globe. These vital components of religious ceremonies, medicine, food, cosmetics, and aphrodisiacs were in great demand and were more costly than precious metals and jewels. Although each region could produce clothing, shelter, and food from the resources in its immediate territory, people of all nations craved rare, exotic odors that literally added spice to their lives and lent an air of mystery to their ceremonies.

The demand for aromatic materials, coupled with their portability, led to the establishment of long distance trade. Fortunately, seeds and herbs could be dried, gums rolled into beads, and fragrances infused in oil or solid perfumes while retaining or improving their properties. This made them extremely portable and relatively impervious to damage.

With trade and the passion for fragrance came adventure and intrigue. Fleets of ships crossed oceans, explorers risked their lives traveling across vast deserts, wars were ignited over land disputes and trade rights, kingdoms were conquered or lost, and love bloomed—all in the pursuit of fragrance. As a result, the quest for fragrance was responsible for molding early world history more than any other single factor.

BABYLONIAN BEGINNINGS

No one knows exactly when trade began, but an import order for cedarwood, myrrh, and cypress was found inscribed on an early Babylonian clay tablet. More than 5,000 years ago, when Egyptians were just learning to

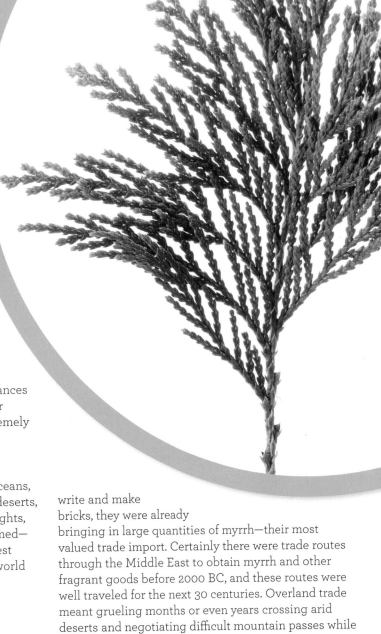

write and make bricks, they were already bringing in large quantities of myrrh—their most valued trade import. Certainly there were trade routes through the Middle East to obtain myrrh and other fragrant goods before 2000 BC, and these routes were well traveled for the next 30 centuries. Overland trade meant grueling months or even years crossing arid deserts and negotiating difficult mountain passes while being threatened by bandits. So aromatics were soon transported by sea, leading to improvements in sailing techniques, vessels, and navigation. Monsoon winds carried double-outrigger canoes along the cinnamon route through the South Seas. Later, Egyptian and eventually Roman traders took advantage of these same winds to take them to India in the summer and home again in the winter.

THE SCENT OF ROYALTY

Wheeling and dealing is not a new art—it was fully employed in the ancient fragrance trade. The great Egyptian Queen Hatshepsut, for one, knew a business opportunity when she saw one. As one of her greatest accomplishments, she sent an expedition to Punt on the African coast to establish what would be a very profitable trade. She also brought back 31 myrrh trees to Egypt, and they were planted in a botanical garden that lined the walkway leading to her massive temple of Deir al-Bahari near Thebes. On the temple walls, the images of the myrrh trees carved in bas-relief can still be seen today.

Other queens made an equal impact on aromatic history. When the Queen of Sheba paid her famous visit to the court of Israel's King Solomon, it was to discuss the fragrance trade. Some sources say she was from southwestern Arabia, the land of frankincense and myrrh, but more likely she was queen of a North Arabian tribe that possibly traded a fragrant resin from the terebinth tree.

Sometimes fragrance simply tagged along in the footsteps of the famous. For example, Alexander the Great's conquests had little to do with the pursuit of fragrant materials. In fact, he despised fragrances because they reminded him of his Persian enemies, and he contemptuously threw out a box of priceless ointments from King Darius' tent after defeating him at the battle of Issos. However, after a few years of traveling through Asia, he became convinced of the joys of fine scent. He anointed his body with fragrant oils and kept incense burning by his throne. And, in his wake, he left the lands he conquered desiring more aromatics.

A WORLD MARKET

Today, cities prosper and fail with the price of oil. So, too, did they in ancient times; however, it was fragrant oils and spices, not fuel oil, that sparked the growth of key cities along the avenues of commerce. With the development of camels as pack animals, the Egyptian city of Alexandria developed into an active trading hub linking several trade routes, including one to distant parts of Arabia.

By the fourth century BC, Babylon had a thriving market, trading in cedar of Lebanon, cypress, pine, fir resin, myrtle, calamus, and juniper. Athens was famous for its hundreds of shops selling scented body oils and solid incense/perfumes. Phoenician merchants dealt in Chinese camphor, Indian cinnamon, black pepper, and sandalwood. Africa, South Arabia, and India supplied lemongrass, ginger, and spikenard, the rhizome of which has an exotic fragrance.

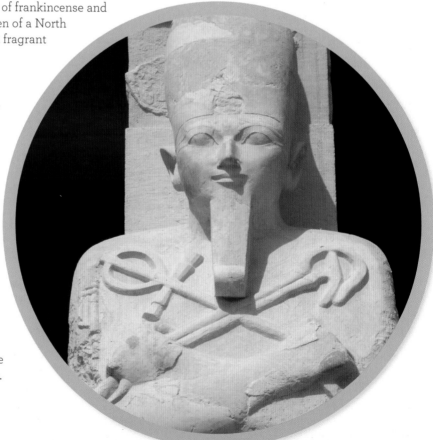

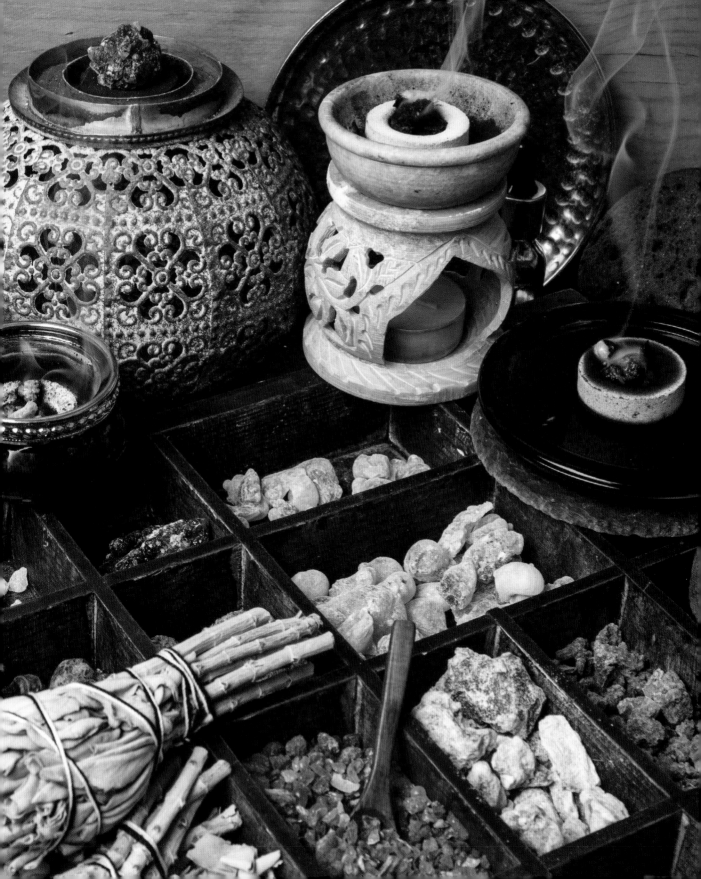

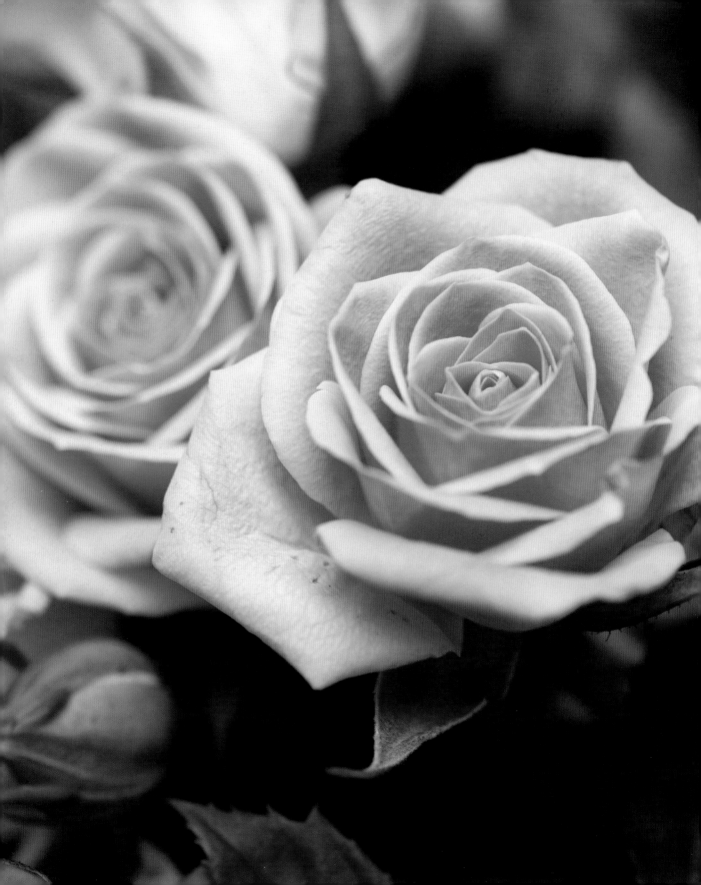

China imported jasmine-scented sesame oil from India and Persia, rose water via the Silk Route, and eventually, Indonesian aromatics: cloves, gum benzoin, ginger, nutmeg, and patchouli. Astute traders knew which locales produced the best oils and fragrances.

REDOLENT WEALTH

Since ancient times, the wealthy and powerful have been able to drown themselves in fragrance. In fact, one unfortunate Roman literally did. He was asphyxiated when the carved ivory ceiling panels in Emperor Nero's dining room slid aside to shower guests, who reclined on floor pillows, with hundreds of pounds of fresh rose petals. In general, wealthy Romans so overindulged themselves in fragrance that the ruler Leptadeni, in 188 BC, issued an edict forbidding such foolish excess.

The Roman population paid little heed to the fragrance prohibition, and demand for incense only increased. By the first century AD, Romans were burning 2,800 tons of imported frankincense and 550 tons of myrrh—both herbs more costly than gold—each year. As a result, Emperor Augustus increased the number of trade ships sailing between Egypt and India fivefold, from twenty to a hundred.

Islamic culture was also rich in fragrance, using it extensively in medicine, cosmetics, and confections. Rose water was mixed into the mortar used to build mosques, and even the ground in paradise was said to emit the scent of musk and saffron. Mohammed himself was once a spice and aromatics merchant who traveled on camel caravans. He loved fragrance, especially rose, mentioning it frequently in his teachings: "Whoever would smell my scent, let him smell the rose."

LINKING EAST AND WEST

Although certainly not the intention, the Crusades of the eleventh, twelfth, and thirteenth centuries acquainted the European population with Arabian ideas and fostered an appreciation of Eastern aromatics, despite repeated warnings by the Christian priesthood that fragrance was associated with Satan. Crusaders returned bearing gifts of oils, fragrant waters, and solid perfumes. Soon the European elite were demanding rose water, and Italians could not live without the addition of orange water to their sweets and confections.

As commerce in fragrance increased between East and West, so did the exchange of ideas. To facilitate trade the Chinese adopted the Indian system of counting. By the eleventh century, Arabs were navigating spice-laden ships from India to China with the Chinese compass and balanced stern rudder. During the next century, the Chinese navy grew from 3,000 to 50,000 sailors to accommodate large vessels that each hauled as much as six thousand baskets of fragrant herbs and spices.

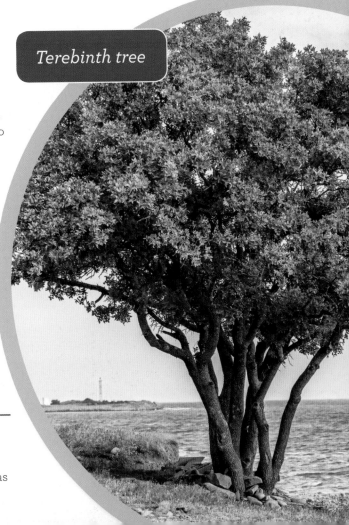

Terebinth tree

China's upper classes were lavish in their use of scent, especially from the seventh century T'ang Dynasty through the Ming Dynasty in the seventeenth century. Everything was scented—baths, clothing, buildings, ink, and paper. Miniature landscapes, in which perfumed smoke escaped from a mountain and coiled around the peak, became the rage.

EXPLORATION AND COLONIZATION

Marco Polo made his famous journey to Kublai Khan's court in the late thirteenth century to establish direct trade between Italy and China. The Italians could thus circumvent Muslim middlemen and their 300 percent markup. The deal was successful, and throughout the thirteenth and fourteenth century Italy monopolized Eastern trade with Europe. Not to be outdone, Spain sent Christopher Columbus across the ocean to seek a shorter route to India.

It was the Portuguese who established a sailing route to India that circumvented Alexandria and Constantinople. In 1498, Vasco de Gama's sailors cheered, "For Christ and spices!" as they reached India, land of fragrant spices and herbs. They brought back so much that nutmegs were said to be rolling in the streets of Lisbon.

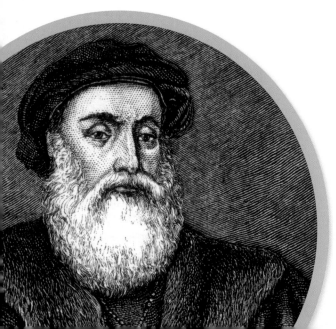

Early in the seventeenth century the Dutch built forts in India, establishing the Dutch East India Company by force. In provinces where they couldn't obtain control, they simply uprooted nutmeg and clove trees so no one else could have them. But the French managed to slip several fragrant plants out from under the Dutch noses. These were planted in the French West Indies and the island of Bourbon (now called Réunion).

INCENSE AND SOLID PERFUMES

For thousands of years and throughout the world, fragrant smoke has purified the air and comforted individuals who were in physical, emotional, or spiritual need. At first, tossing a few fragrant plant twigs into the fire served the purpose, but eventually solid incense was created using ground gums and plants mixed with honey. These were formed into solid cubes and set on a coal from the fire. In many cultures, elaborate ceremonial burners were designed to hold cubes of incense atop smoldering coals.

PURIFICATION

The ancients filled temples, council rooms, and homes with incense, using it even more liberally than we would an air freshener. Small wonder, since incense was able to dispel the disagreeable smells of unsanitary living conditions. In Europe, Arabia, India, China, and throughout North America, dwellings were fumigated to drive out the evil spirits that were believed to cause illness while, at the same time, ridding the dwelling of fleas and bugs. During epidemics, people who flocked to temples and churches were probably helped by the burning of antiseptic herbs. Hippocrates, the father of medicine, is said to have freed Athens from the plague by burning aromatic plants. Respiratory and rheumatic ills, headaches, unconsciousness, and other medical problems were treated by breathing in smoke arising from aromatic plants. And sometimes wet, aromatic herbs or herb teas were dropped on hot rocks to create a steam that was inhaled. Both techniques proved effective in treating sinus congestion, lung problems, or earache.

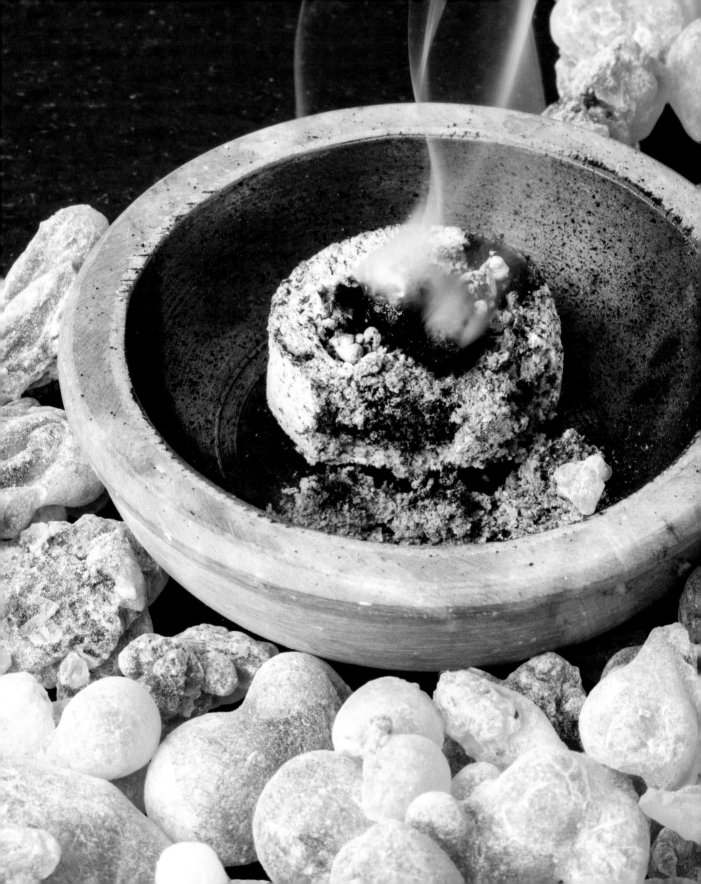

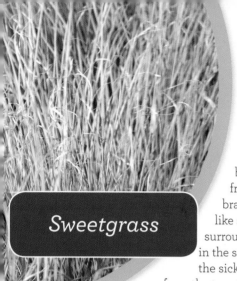

Sweetgrass

During religious and healing ceremonies, Native Americans burned tight bundles of fragrant herbs and braids of vanilla-like sweetgrass and surrounded themselves in the smoke. And to heal the sick, rocks steaming from the tea of goldenrod, fleabane, pearly everlasting, and echinacea were placed next to a patient, and both were covered with hides or blankets to make a type of aroma-filled mini-sauna.

VERSATILE *ARÓMATA*

Throughout Europe, Arabia, and India, incense proved to be immensely versatile; it was used as perfume, medicine, and even mouthwash. Remember, early incense contained nothing other than ground herbs, plant gums, and even honey. (Only much later was messy charcoal and inedible saltpeter added so that, once ignited, the incense would continue burning.) Since most of the herbs were highly antiseptic, when rubbed on the skin and melted by body heat, they released a scent and disinfected wounds. Incense was even ingested as medicine. It is no surprise, then, that the Greek word *arómata* had several meanings: incense, perfume, spice, and aromatic medicine. The Chinese also had one word, *heang*, to describe perfume, incense, and the concept of fragrance.

Some aromatics were even found to help with weight loss, digestion, or menstrual regularity. Rome's most famous perfume, *Susinon*, was a diuretic when ingested. It relieved various types of inflammation. *Amarakinon* treated indigestion and hemorrhoids and encouraged menstruation, either when ingested or when applied directly to the affliction. It was also worn as perfume. Spikenard was the main ingredient in another perfume that could be sucked as a throat lozenge to relieve coughs and laryngitis.

AN INTOXICATION OF MIND AND EMOTIONS

Throughout the world, incense has been employed to affect mind and emotions. According to the Japanese, it opens us to the transcendent, purifies mind and body, keeps you alert, acts as a companion in solitude, and brings moments of peace amidst busy affairs. The fragrant smoke billowing from Chinese bronze incense burners was classified into six basic moods: tranquil, reclusive, luxurious, beautiful, refined, and noble.

Certain plants have been burned for their intoxicating or aphrodisiac properties. In Delphi, Greece, the oracle priestesses sat on stools over holes in the floor that emitted fumes of bay leaves to inspire visions. While little of Delphi's grandeur remains today, you can still see the hidden incense chamber underneath the floor. Women in Tibet called *dainyals* held cloths over their heads to capture cedar smoke, which would send them into prophetic chanting. Aromatic plants with hypnotic properties were used similarly by Australian aborigines and by Native Americans.

Cleopatra used scent to lure Mark Anthony. Her slaves fanned incense smoke onto the sails of her ship. In *Anthony and Cleopatra*, Shakespeare describes these sails as "so perfumed that the winds were love-sick with them." This was probably not far from the truth, since the scent she chose is thought to be that of the delicious camphire (henna) mentioned in the Song of Solomon—long regarded as an aphrodisiac.

RELIGIOUS USES OF INCENSE

In nearly every culture, incense was believed to attract the gods and goddesses, keep evil spirits at bay, and purify body and soul. Ancient peoples, believing that spirit and life entered the body through their breath, also thought that inhaling certain odors brought them closer to God. Fragrance was considered akin to the divine because it was invisible, mysterious, and attractive. They called aroma the soul of the plant and believed it was a gift from God. They also believed that the deities would find prayers—breathed into the smoke which carried them aloft—more pleasing when sweetly scented.

Its association with pagan sensuality and its excessive use by the Arabs, Romans, and Jews gave incense a bad name among the majority of early Christians. However, some sects did use it exclusively for religious ceremonies. Gnostic Christians from the first to the fourth centuries were deeply influenced by Egyptian philosophy and adopted the ancient belief that a plant's fragrance is associated with the soul of man. Eventually, the Catholic Church embraced the use of incense to purify and bless their statues, relics, altars, and those participating in the mass.

To the Chinese Taoists, fragrance also held a religious significance. Among the 10,000 rites of Taoist Buddhism, it is said that the "burning of incense has primacy," representing the soul's liberation from limitations of the material world. To enhance their experience, they sometimes incorporated psychoactive plants such as cannabis into their incense. The incense burner itself, called *fa lu*, became an object of worship.

THE ART AND PRACTICE OF SCENT

Although the Japanese came relatively late to the use of incense, they quickly developed it into a sophisticated art called *koh-do* that was taught in special schools. Still practiced by a few people today, participants in the incense ceremony had to bathe and dress in clean clothes so that they carried no odors into the room. They then tried to guess the different characteristics of the incense. The winner went home with a prize.

The world's first novel, *Prince Genji*, written by Lady Murasaki Shikibu in the eleventh century, describes the practice of scenting one's kimono sleeves. Small incense burners were "held for a moment inside each sleeve" so

that scent floated about whenever a motion was made by the hand. Japan's earliest anthology of poems refers to this practice:

In the moonlight
Where are the plum blossoms?
Let their fragrance guide you.
The fragrance—
More alluring than the color—
Whose scented sleeves have brushed
The blossoms in my garden?

—From the *Kokinshu*

The European elite also scented their sleeves. Ladies of the court pinned scented pendants that held solid perfumes imported from Arabia into the sleeves of their cut-velvet gowns. They also kept the perfume in lockets worn around the neck where they could be conveniently sniffed. Orange blossom oil was extracted and combined with pressed almond pulp to make the very popular perfume ointment pomades. *Pomme d'ambre*, on the other hand, were scented balls of ambergris, spices, honey, and wine that hung from the belt in a small, perforated container. Even the slightest movement of a skirt would surround one in fragrance.

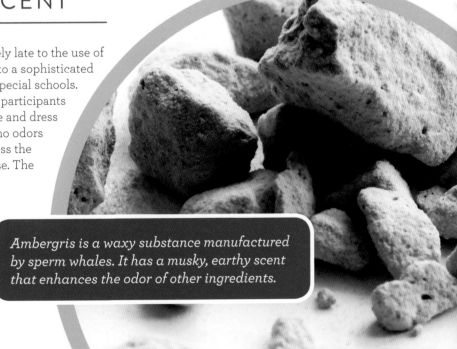

Ambergris is a waxy substance manufactured by sperm whales. It has a musky, earthy scent that enhances the odor of other ingredients.

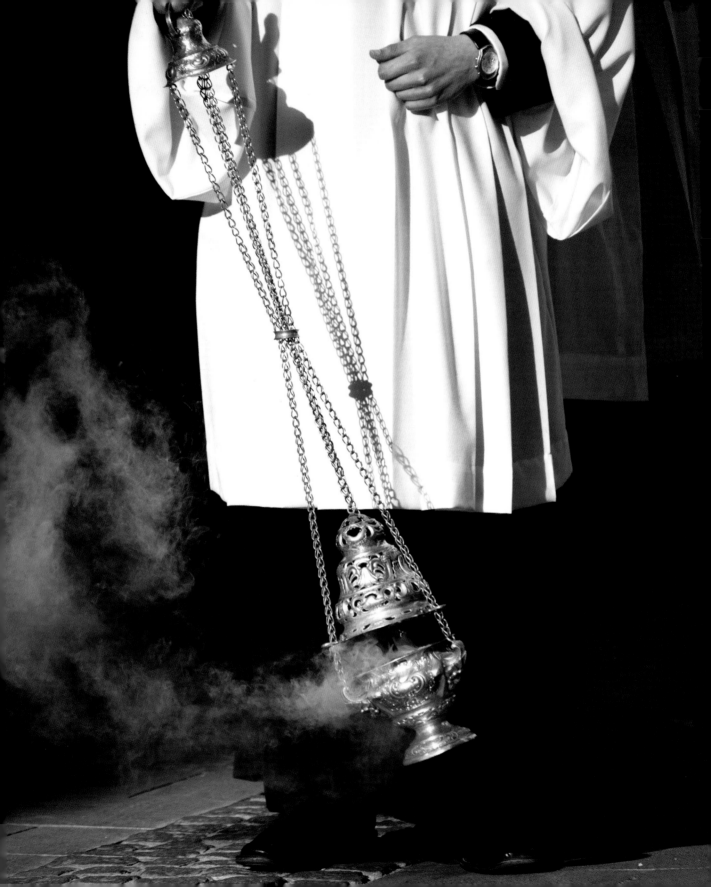

BODY OILS

Fragrance also found its way into religious and secular life via scented oils. These were made, as they still are today, by extracting plant oils into fat or vegetable oil and then straining out the used plant material. They were used liberally in religious ceremonies to consecrate temples, alters, statues, candles, and priests.

RELIGIOUS USE OF FRAGRANT OILS

The Book of Exodus (30:22–25) provides one of the earliest recipes for an anointing oil—given by God to Moses to be used in the initiation of priests. The ingredients included myrrh, cinnamon, calamus, and cassia blended into olive oil.

When Mary Magdalene anointed Christ's feet and wiped them with her hair, it was with an oil made from costly spikenard. The name Christ, or Christos, from the Greek *chriein*, literally means "to anoint," and the frankincense and myrrh brought by the wise men to the Christ child most likely were anointing oils. These oils were considered to be more valuable than the gold that was carried by the third wise man.

ANCIENT EGYPTIAN SCENTS

Egyptian talent for formulating scented oils became legendary, and their oils were certainly potent: Calcite pots filled with richly scented oils still held a faint odor when King Tutankamen's tomb was opened 3,000 years later. Egyptians were especially creative with the use of scent and did not restrict it to religious rites. An individual's special odor, or *khaibt,* was represented by a hieroglyph of a fan and was thought capable of influencing the emotions of others.

The first beauty spa may have been the perfume factory owned by Cleopatra at En Gedi, by the Dead Sea. Individuals were apparently offered health and beauty treatments, since the ruins of the factory show seats in what are believed to have been waiting and treatment rooms. Fragrant herbs were blended into specially prepared olive oil. Unfortunately, the book in which Cleopatra recorded recipes for her body oils, *Cleopatra Gynaeciarum Libri*, is long lost. We know of it only through its mention in Roman texts.

BATHED IN FRAGRANCE

The Romans, who did not enjoy the messy process of infusing and straining scented oils, imported most of theirs from Egypt. Men and women alike literally bathed in fragrance. So prevalent was the use of scent that Romans affectionately called their sweethearts "my myrrh, my cinnamon," just as today we call our loved ones "honey."

The Greeks were especially attracted to the use of scented oils. In fact, Hippocrates recommended the use of body oils in the bath. In Athens, proprietors of *unguentarii* shops sold marjoram, lily, thyme, sage, anise, rose, and iris infused in oil and thickened with beeswax. They packaged their unguents (from a word meaning to smear or anoint) in small, elaborately decorated ceramic pots, as they still do today. However, in those times the shopkeepers were consulted as doctors, and their products were sold for a multitude of medicinal uses.

Greek men and women anointed their bodies for both personal enhancement and sensuality. The men used a different scented oil, chosen for its particular attributes, for each part of their body. Most of the oils they used, such as mint for the arms, were warm and stimulating. Oils were also used to massage tight muscles. Athletes in India, on the Mediterranean island of Crete, and later in Greece and Rome, had specially prepared oils rubbed into their muscles before, and often after, participating in their athletic games.

East Indian Tantric practice turned women into a veritable garden of earthly delights. They anointed themselves with jasmine on their hands, patchouli on the neck and cheeks, amber on their breasts, spikenard in the hair, musk on the abdomen, sandalwood on the thighs, and saffron on their feet. Men, however, applied only sandalwood to their own bodies.

The daily bathing ritual in India required the application of sesame oils scented with jasmine, coriander, cardamom, basil, costus, pandanus, agarwood, pine, saffron, champac, and clove. Ancient Vedic religious and medical books gave instruction on balancing body temperature, temperament, and digestion with such aromas, and some of their therapeutic uses were certainly passed on to the West.

In Egypt, everyone used body oils, from royalty to laborers. Builders constructing a burial site went on strike in the twelfth century BC not just because the food was bad, but even worse, they complained, "We have no ointment." They depended upon the oils to ease sore muscles after a day of hauling and carving huge stones and to protect their skin from the intense Egyptian sun.

Throughout the Americas, massage with scented oils was also used as therapy and was often the first treatment given. One massage oil prepared by the Incas contained valerian and other relaxing herbs that were thickened with seaweed. The Aztecs massaged the sick with scented ointments in their sweat lodges.

PERFUME

Perfume as we know it today—packaged in tiny, expensive bottles with a high alcohol content and hundreds of chemical compounds—is a relatively new invention.

MARIA PROPHETISSA'S INVENTION

The first written description of a distiller to produce essential oils appears around the first century AD. Maria Prophetissa, known as Mary the Jewess, invented a mechanism that looked something like a double-boiler. She described the essential oil it produced as an "angel

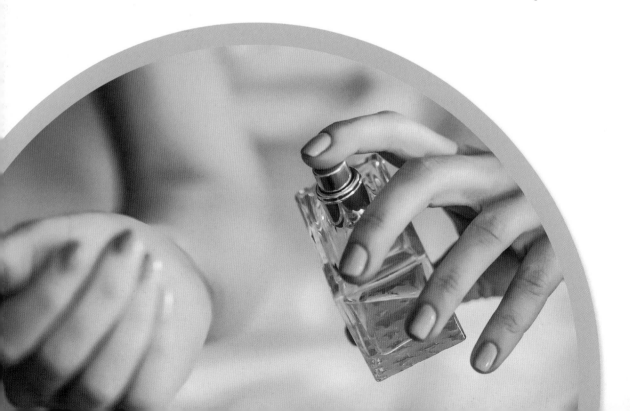

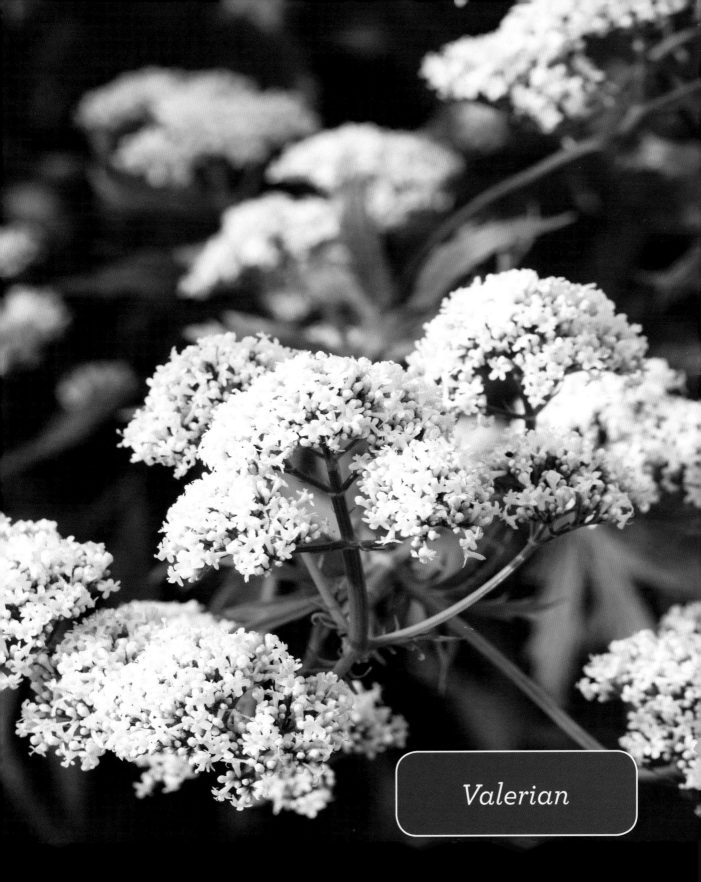

Valerian

who descends from the sky." By the second century, the Chinese and Arabs were distilling essential oils, and Japan followed suit a few centuries later.

Prophetissa's inventions could also distill alcohol. Combining it with essential oils and diluting it with water produced a new type of fragrance. These scented "waters" made the body smell sweet and also acted as medicine and cosmetics. When dabbed on the skin, they improved skin tone and diminished blemishes. When taken internally, they relieved indigestion, soothed menstrual cramps, or treated myriad other ailments. Thus was born the "medicinal tonic."

AROMATIC WATERS

If you have ever appreciated a fine European liquor such as Benedictine or Fra Angelica, you are benefiting from the stills of early monastery infirmaries and herbariums. Many monks and nuns were dedicated herbalists who served as both doctor and pharmacist to their patients. Aromatic waters were one of their favorite prescriptions.

Some sources credit the twelfth century herbalist Saint Hildegard, Abbess of Bingen, with inventing lavender water, which she mentions in a treatise on medicinal and aromatic herbs. However it originated, this aromatic water took Europe by storm. By the fourteenth century, lavender water was so popular that the French King Charles V had lavender planted in the gardens at the Louvre to ensure the supply.

Another famous monastic concoction was *Aqua Mirabilis*, or "Miracle Water," a water and alcohol combination spiked with essential oils. It was sipped to improve vision and to treat rheumatic pain, fever, and congestion; it was also said to improve memory and reduce melancholy. In addition, it was splashed on the body to improve one's smell.

Carmelite Water was prepared by European Carmelite nuns from a secret formula that we now know included melissa (lemon balm) and angelica. It aided both digestion and the complexion, depending upon its use. Modern versions of Miracle Water and Carmelite Water are still sold in Europe today.

EAU DE COLOGNE

In 1732, aromatic waters were further refined into cologne when Giovanni Maria Farina of Cologne, France, took over his uncle's business. *Aqua Admirabilis*, a blend of neroli, bergamot, lavender, and rosemary in grape alcohol, which has a distinct fruity scent, was used on the face and also treated sore gums and indigestion. Soldiers dubbed it "Eau de Cologne," meaning Cologne water, after the town, and the name cologne stuck to all perfumed waters since then. The rumor was that Napoleon went through several bottles a day, an endorsement that made the cologne so popular that 39 nearly identical products were created. A half-century of lawsuits against these illegal knock-off colognes followed. After four centuries as the undisputed favorite, Queen of Hungary Water was displaced by Eau de Cologne as the fragrance in most demand.

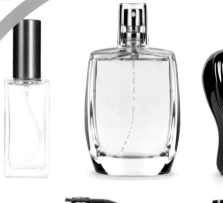
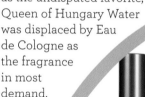
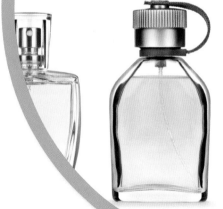

CHEMISTRY AND COSMETICS

A little more than 100 years ago, the fragrance industry was suddenly thrust into the modern chemical age. Previously, cologne and even soap had always been considered part of the medicinal pharmacy. Then, in 1867, the Paris International Exhibition boldly exhibited them in a separate section dubbed cosmetics. This radical move birthed an entirely new industry that paved the way for a new product: perfume.

The very next year, the first commercial synthetic essential oil was developed in the laboratory. With its fresh smell of newly mowed hay, the synthetic oil was an instant hit with cologne manufacturers. Thousands of synthetic fragrances, even those imitating the rarest and most expensive essential oils, were engineered mostly from petroleum chemicals.

These synthetic oils changed the character of personal fragrance forever. The new chemicals were so concentrated, they allowed the manufacture of powerful perfumes. Replacing light colognes that were liberally splashed on, just a few small drops of perfume completely scented an individual. Still other newly-invented chemical additives made that scent linger for hours. Of course, with all the synthetic ingredients, colognes, and perfumes were no longer medicinal—and certainly not edible. For the first time in history, they were purely a cosmetic product.

Promoted by the newly emerging fashion design world, major perfume houses such as Guerlain, Bourjois, and Rimmel established themselves in France. While the Victorian era had frowned on anything but the lightest scents, styles changed when American soldiers returned from France following World War I, laden with gifts of perfume. The idea of wearing a personal fragrance caught on.

AROMATHERAPY COMES OF AGE

Today, perfume, food, medicine, and aromatherapy products are viewed as separate entities, although aromatherapy is slowly reclaiming its medicinal heritage. A French chemist, René-Maurice Gattefossé, coined the term *aromatherapie* in 1928. His family were perfumers, but his interest in the therapeutic use of essential oils began when he severely burned his hand in a laboratory explosion. He deliberately plunged his hand into a nearby container of lavender oil to ease the pain, and was amazed at how quickly it healed. He wrote numerous books and papers on the chemistry of perfume and cosmetics. Around the same time another Frenchman, Albert Couvreur, published a book on the medicinal uses of essential oils.

A new wave of aromatherapist practitioners was inspired by this work, one of whom was Dr. Jean Valnet, who, while an army surgeon during World War II, used essential oils such as thyme, clove, lemon, and chamomile on wounds and burns. He later used essential oils to treat psychiatric problems. Marguerite Maury, a French biochemist, developed therapeutic methods for applying these oils to the skin as a massage, reintroducing an ancient method of aromatherapy to the modern world.

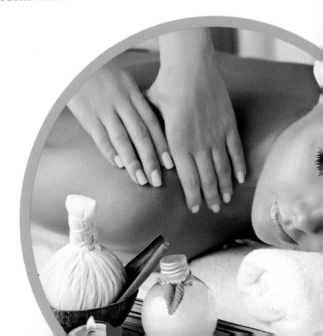

THE ESSENCE OF THE SUBJECT

Remember the penetrating fragrance of an herb or flower garden on a hot summer's day, or the crisp smell of an orange as you peel it? These odors are the fragrance of the plant's essential oils, the potent, volatile, and aromatic substance contained in various parts of the plant, including its flowers, leaves, roots, wood, seeds, fruit, and bark. The essential oils carry concentrations of the plant's healing properties—those same properties that traditional Western medicine utilizes in many drugs.

AROMATHERAPY

Aromatherapy simply means the application of those healing powers—it is a fragrant cure. Professional aromatherapists focus very specifically on the controlled use of essential oils to treat ailments and disease and to promote physical and emotional well-being.

Aromatherapy doesn't just work through the sense of smell alone, however. Inhalation is only one application method. Essential oils can also be diluted in a carrier oil and applied to the skin. When used topically, the oils penetrate the skin, taking direct action on body tissues and organs in the vicinity of application. They also enter the bloodstream and are carried throughout the body. Of course, when applied topically the fragrance of the essential oil is also inhaled.

There are three different modes of action in the body: pharmacological, which affects the chemistry of the body; physiological, which affects the ability of the body to function and process; and psychological, which affects emotions and attitudes. These three modes interact continuously. Aromatherapy is so powerful partly because it affects all three modes. You choose the application method based on where you most want the effects concentrated and on what is most convenient and pleasing to you.

Aromatherapy is actually an aspect of a larger category of healing treatment known as herbal medicine. Herbal medicine also utilizes the healing powers of plants to treat physical and emotional problems, but it uses the whole plant or parts of the plant, such as leaves, flowers, roots, and seeds, rather than the essential oil. Aromatherapy and herbal medicine can be used individually, or they can be used jointly to augment potential healing benefits.

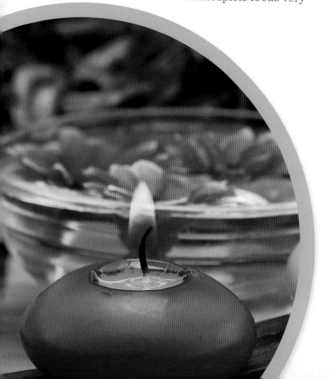

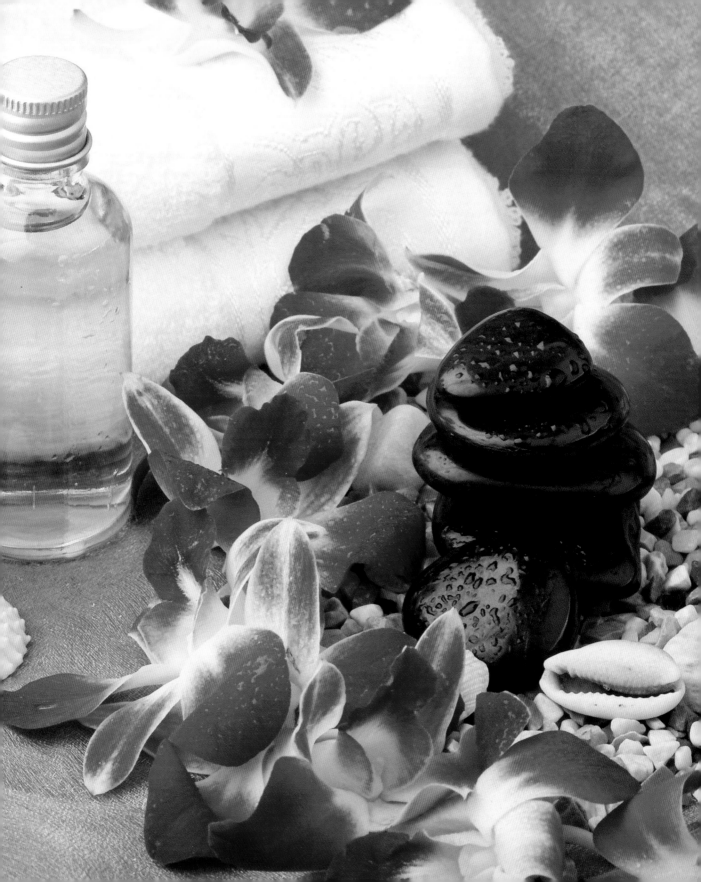

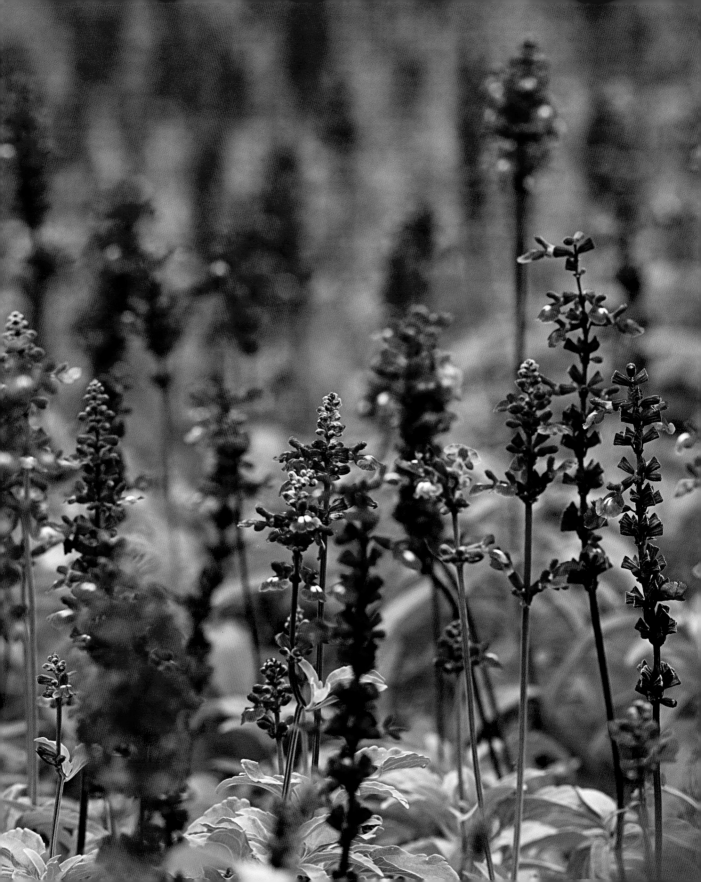

THERAPEUTIC USES OF ESSENTIAL OILS

You can treat a wide range of physical problems with aromatherapy. Almost all essential oils have antiseptic properties and are able to fight infection and destroy bacteria, fungi, yeast, parasites, and/or viruses. Many essential oils also reduce aches and pain, soothe or rout inflammations and spasms, stimulate the immune system and insulin and hormone production, affect blood circulation, dissolve mucus and open nasal passages, or aid digestion—just to mention a few of their amazing properties. For the purposes of this book, we will consider basic beauty care as a therapeutic treatment that helps establish well-being. For instance, using aromatherapy in cosmetics and skin preparations can help counter external problems such as skin infections and eczema. It simply depends on which essential oils you use and how you use them.

Aromatherapy can also have a considerable influence on our emotions. Sniffing clary sage, for example, can quell panic, while the fragrance released by peeling an orange can make you feel more optimistic. Since your mind strongly influences your health and is itself a powerful healing tool, it makes aromatherapy's potential even more exciting.

Many essential oils perform more than one function, so having just a half-dozen or so on hand will help you treat a wide range of common physical ailments and emotional problems. The beauty of aromatherapy is that you can create a blend of oils that will benefit both in one treatment. For example, you can blend a combination of essential oils that not only stops indigestion, but also reduces the nervous condition that encouraged it. Or, you could design an aromatherapy body lotion that both improves your complexion and relieves depression.

THE ESSENCE OF ESSENTIAL OILS

Plants take the light of the sun, the minerals of the earth, and the carbon dioxide exhaled by humans and animals and, through photosynthesis, transform them into the building blocks of medicine. Among the most important therapeutic compounds manufactured by plants are essential oils. These volatile substances contain a variety of active constituents and are also responsible for each plant's unique fragrance.

FRAGRANCE MOLECULES

The basic elements of carbon, hydrogen, and oxygen combine to form the different organic molecular compounds that produce aromas. So far, more than 30,000 of these molecular compounds have been

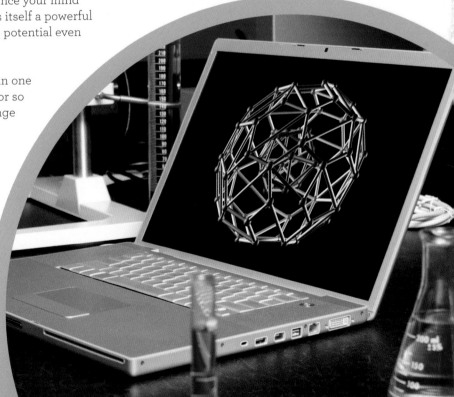

identified and named. Most individual essential oils consist of many different aromatic molecular compounds. In fact, the essential oil from just one plant may contain as many as one hundred different fragrance molecules. In nature there are thousands of plants, all with unique fragrances that are comprised of different combinations of these molecules.

Plants that smell similar to one another usually contain some of the same molecular compounds. Lemon verbena, lemon balm (melissa), lemon thyme, lemon eucalyptus, citronella, lemongrass, and lemon itself, for instance, all smell like lemon because they contain a lemon-scented molecule called citral. But it is the other aromatic molecules they contain that give each plant its unique fragrance.

Aromatic compounds are grouped under larger classes of compounds such as terpenes, phenols, aldehydes, alcohols, ketones, acids, esters, coumarins, and occasionally, oxides. Citral is an aldehyde; eugenol is a phenol. Each molecular compound has characteristic scents and actions on the body. Some may be cooling and relaxing, while others are warming and stimulating. Some are better for treating indigestion, while others are antiseptic.

Every effect of an essential oil has a chemical explanation. These effects include their biological activity in the body (beneficial, irritating, or toxic), their solubility (in oil or alcohol, for instance), how rapidly they evaporate in air or are absorbed through the skin, and how well different oils combine as scents. Aldehydes such as those found in cinnamon and lemongrass, for example, have a slightly fruity odor and may often cause skin irritation and allergic reaction. Ketones found in fennel, caraway, and rosemary are not metabolized easily and may pass unchanged into the urine. The phenols found in clove and thyme are very likely to be irritating.

The proportion of aromatic compounds in a particular type of plant is not necessarily constant. This proportion can change from year to year depending on the plants's growing conditions, including geographic location, elevation, climate, soil quality, and the methods used to harvest it and extract the essential oil. Consistent variations found in the same species are called chemotypes, or chemical types (CT). Aromatherapists often take advantage of these natural alterations, selecting a certain chemotype over the standard for its special attributes.

THE PHYSIOLOGY OF SCENT

Essential oil molecules enter the body through the nose and skin. Since these molecules are extremely small and float easily through the air, you can simply inhale them into your lungs, which then disperse them into your bloodstream. The blood quickly carries them throughout your body. Essential oil molecules are also small enough to be absorbed through the pores of the skin. Once absorbed, some molecules can enter the bloodstream, while others remain in the area of application or evaporate into the air. How much goes where depends on the size of the essential oil molecules, the method of application (massage increases absorption), and the carrier containing the essential oil, be it alcohol, vegetable oil, vinegar, or water. This makes essential oils perfect for healing a specific skin problem as well as the entire body.

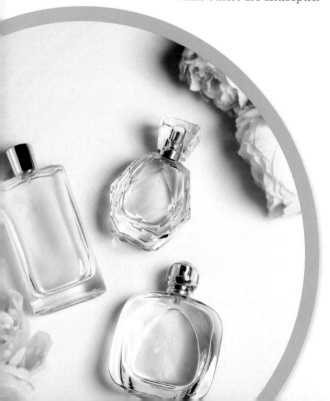

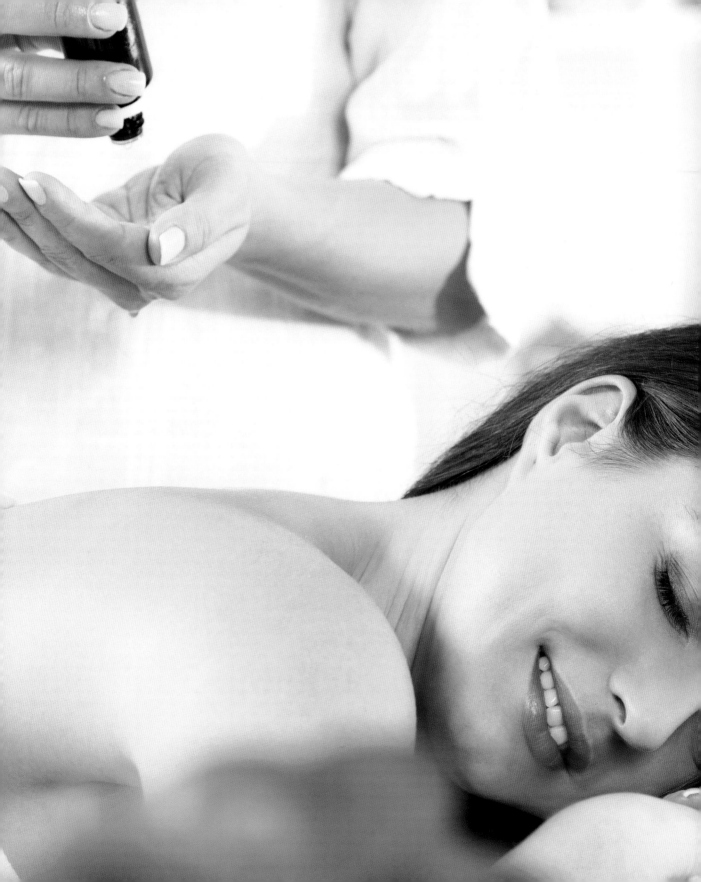

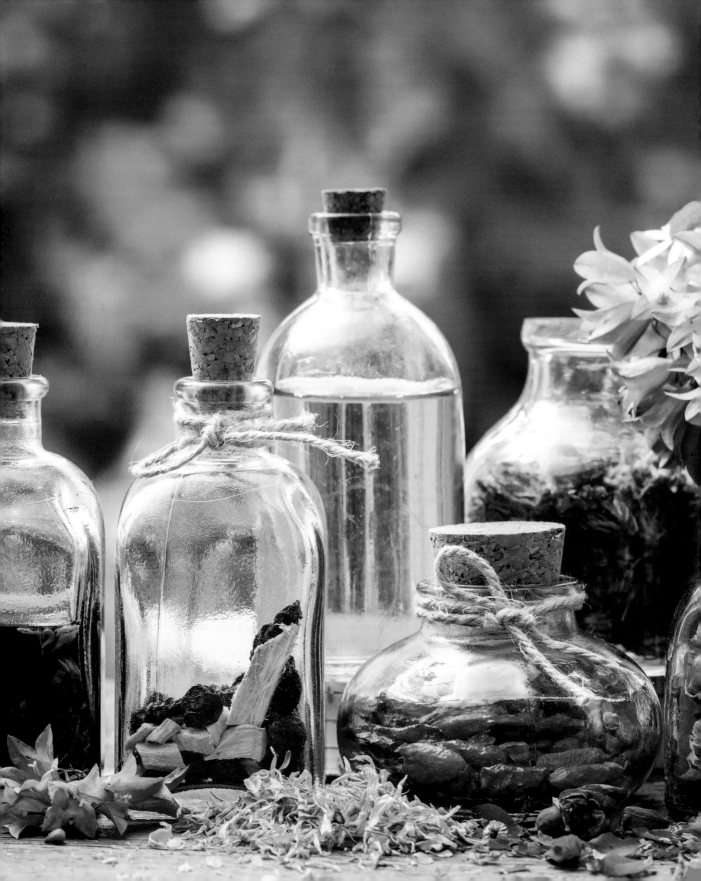

The sense of smell has its own important mechanisms. High in the nose is the olfactory epithelium, two smell receptors about the size of dimes. The receptors pick up volatile and lipid-soluble molecules using tiny filaments called cilia, which may actually be able to identify odor molecules by their "shape." It is believed that these odor receptors are coded by a huge family of genes to sense particular components of smell that produce a characteristic "fingerprint" pattern of activity in the brain.

From the olfactory mucus membrane, signals travel to olfactory bulbs that extend forward like tiny spoons from the brain. An electrical impulse then goes directly to the limbic system, which is part of what is called the primitive or "old" brain. Smell, it seems, was our first sense, and our old brain actually evolved from the olfactory stalks. Because recognition of smell moves directly into the old brain, it completely bypasses areas that control reasoning and the central nervous system. Thus, it directly influences survival mechanisms such as "fight or flight" reactions and the autonomic functions of the body, including heartbeat, body temperature, appetite, digestion, sexual arousal, and memory—the functions we can't control by will or reason. It also affects instincts such as emotions, attraction/repulsion, lust, and creativity. The senses of hearing and vision, by contrast, first stimulate the thalamus, which registers only warmth and pain. Furthermore, the old brain is directly connected to the hypothalamus and pituitary glands, and therefore to our immune system and hormones, which is why smell affects them so powerfully.

Damage to the limbic system of the old brain has been found to adversely affect memory and cause eating disorders and sexual dysfunction. Thus, medical researchers hope to someday treat such memory disorders as Alzheimer disease with fragrance. Other treatments being researched include those for fatigue, migraine headaches, food cravings, depression, schizophrenia, and anxiety.

ESSENTIAL OILS AND OUR DAILY LIVES

Have you ever smelled a certain flower or cologne and suddenly experienced déjà vu? Or perhaps you've caught a whiff of fir and immediately envisioned a Christmas tree even in the middle of July. Scent can transport us back to previous experiences, triggering long forgotten feelings associated with those memories. That's because a particular aroma triggers areas of the brain that influence your emotions, memory, cardiovascular functioning, and hormonal balance. Your body thinks you are there!

In fact, memories associated with scent influence us more than most of us realize. Realtors know that the smell of baking cookies, heightened by the

MEDICINAL PROPERTIES OF AROMATIC COMPOUNDS

Terpenes and Sesquiterpenes: antiseptic, anti-inflammatory, carminative, and stimulating. Found in a majority of essential oils, including citruses, flowers, leaves, seeds, roots, and woods. Essential oils in this group: cardamom, carrot seed, cypress, ginger, grapefruit, sandalwood, spikenard, patchouli.

Phenols: stimulating, strongly antibacterial, can be skin irritants. Essential oils in this group: clove, oregano, savory, some thymes.

Aldehydes: calming, sedating, antiseptic, anti-inflammatory, popular perfume aromatics. Essential oils in this group: cinnamon, cumin, lemon scents.

Alcohols: toning, energizing, antibacterial, antiviral, with pleasant, uplifting fragrances. Essential oils in this group: geranium, rosewood, petitgrain, rose, tea tree.

Ketones: dissolves mucus and fats, heals wounds, includes some toxic factors. Essential oils in this group: sage, hyssop, jasmine, fennel, peppermint.

Acids: anti-inflammatory, antiseptic, moisturizing. Mostly found in combination with alcohols to create esters. Essential oils in this group: birch, rosewood, niaouli.

Esters: balancing, relaxing, soothing, antispasmodic, antifungal, with fruity aromas. Essential oils in this group: lavender, bergamot, clary sage, ylang ylang, neroli, Roman chamomile, marjoram.

Coumarins: calming and uplifting, blood thinning, photosensitizing, some toxic properties. Essential oils in this group: bergamot, angelica, citruses.

Oxides: expectorant. Essential oils in this group: eucalyptus, bay, hyssop.

aroma of vanilla, can sell a house because it reminds potential buyers of being nurtured. In fact, realtors can skip the baking cookies and simply scent the air with a vanilla fragrance.

THE SWEET SMELL OF SUCCESS

Studies have proven that certain scents summon deep-seated memories and affect personality, behavior, and sleep patterns. They have demonstrated that pleasant smells put people into better moods and make them more willing to negotiate, cooperate, and compromise.

As a result, several large Tokyo corporations began circulating the essential oils of lemon, peppermint, and cypress through their ventilation systems to keep workers alert and attentive on the job. As a happy side effect, this practice is said to reduce the employees' urge to smoke. Pleasing fragrances are being pumped into offices, stores, and hotels in cities around the world to make the atmosphere more relaxing and invigorating, a task that multidimensional essential oils handle with ease. Of course, what these companies really want is for you to feel so comfortable that you will stay longer and return often.

NATURAL UPPERS AND DOWNERS

Memory and association are only one way scents affect us psychologically. According to researchers studying aromacology, the science of medicinal aromas, fragrance actually alters our brain waves.

For instance, stimulating scents such as peppermint and eucalyptus intensify brain waves, making the mind sharper and clearer. The effects are similar to those of coffee, but are achieved without caffeine's detrimental impact on the adrenal glands. As a result, aroma is currently helping workers such as truck drivers and air traffic controllers, whose jobs—and the safety of others—depend on their being attentive.

Certain fragrances can also produce the opposite effect. If you inhale a flowery draft of chamomile tea, your brain waves will lengthen, causing you to feel relaxed. This is similar to the effect of taking a sedative drug but without the concomitant liver damage. Some essential oils have effects similar to antidepressant drugs, according to the Olfaction Research Group at Warwick University in England. Italian psychiatrist Paolo Rovesti, M.D., helped his patients overcome depression using the scents of various citruses, such as orange, bergamot, lemon, and lemon verbena.

Psychologists help people overcome anxiety, tension, and mood swings by having them associate a scent with feelings of rest and contentment. The psychologist uses biofeedback or visualization techniques to help the client relax, and then sniff a relaxing scent. Later, the client can simply smell the relaxation scent when he or she becomes nervous or anxious.

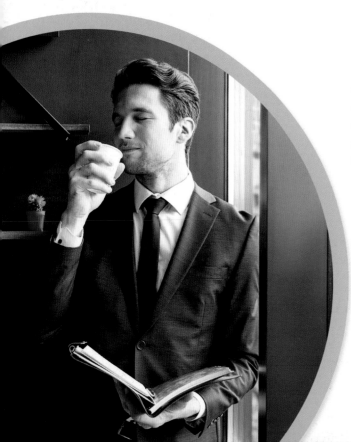

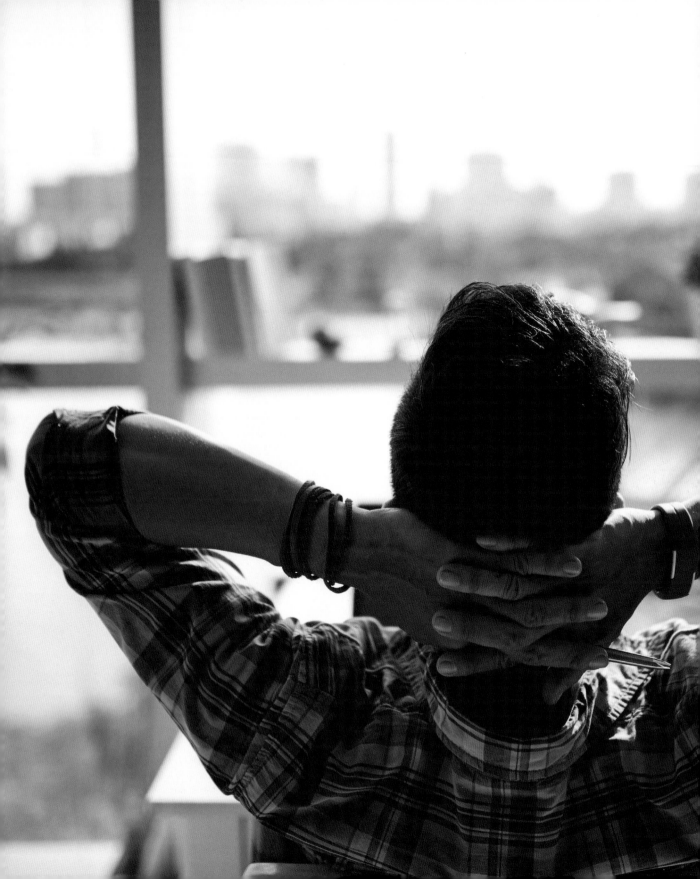

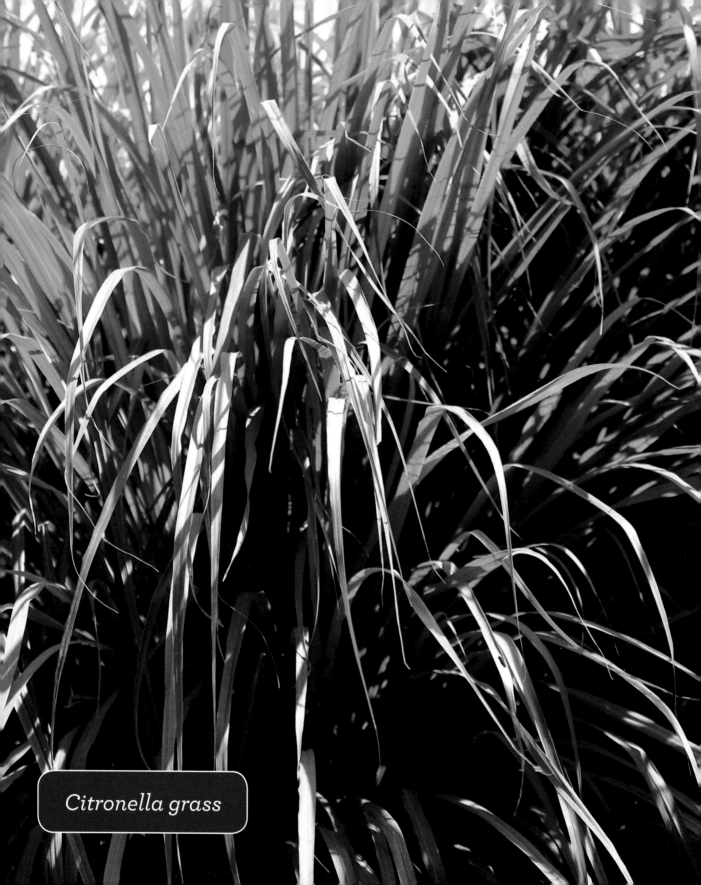

Citronella grass

RESPECT YOUR PLANT ALLIES

Essential oils can be purchased in health stores, some grocery stores, and of course online. Their easy availability and the fact that they are distilled directly from plants may make cautionary guidelines seem unnecessary—after all, there are no FDA warnings or lists of side effects on their labels—but you should *never* underestimate the capacity this natural pharmacy has for both beneficial and harmful results. Essential oils contain powerful chemical compounds. Misuse via direct topical application or ingestion can result in serious harm.

Even when using essential oils via diffusion, consider the dilution rate and size of the room. Can the oils disperse readily? How long will the exposure be? Prolonged exposure (over one hour) to relatively high levels of essential oil vapor may lead to nausea, headache, or feeling "spaced out." If you find yourself feeling like this, get some fresh air right away. Brief exposure is better.

Infants and toddlers are more sensitive to the potency of essential oils. What's safe and pleasant for adults may be overwhelming for young children.

You should never ingest essential oils. There are some instances where practitioners will recommend the ingestion of small, diluted amounts to address specific conditions, but you should never do this without the guidance of a qualified professional.

When applying essential oils to the skin, always dilute them with a carrier oil (more on carrier oils later). As you increase the ratio of essential oil to carrier oil, you run a greater risk of an adverse dermal reaction. Higher levels of essential oils also increase the risk of **sensitization** occurring. For this reason, most aromatherapists do not recommend direct (neat) application of undiluted essential oils to the skin.

SENSITIZATION

Another reason for diluting essential oils and applying them topically only in small quantities is the risk of sensitization. This allergic reaction can occur when the skin is first exposed to an essential oil. The effect on the skin may not be noticeable at first, but repeated exposure eventually creates an inflammatory reaction. The reaction may manifest as blotchiness or redness. Once sensitization occurs, the individual may remain sensitive to the substance for years.

While many oils are generally well-tolerated by most individuals when applied via massage in a carrier oil, others are best avoided. Be especially careful with the following essential oils (or avoid them entirely), as they are known to be dermal irritants:

BASIL
BAY
BENZOIN
BIRCH
CINNAMON BARK OR LEAF
CITRONELLA
CLOVE BUD
CUMIN
GINGER
LEMONGRASS
LEMON VERBENA
OREGANO
TAGETES
THYME

This is a partial list. Remember: everyone has different sensitivities. More and more essential oils are being made available commercially each year, and the effects of some are not well understood.

Rubbing just a few drops of most essential oils directly onto the skin could easily amount to ingesting the equivalent of 10 cups of herb tea all at once! In addition to irritating or even burning your skin, you could damage your liver and kidneys, which must detoxify large amounts of essential oils once they enter the blood stream.

PHOTOSENSITIZATION

Some essential oils act as photosensitizers. Reactions may range from mild color change and irritation to extreme burning. If you have used photosensitizing essential oils topically, avoid prolonged exposure to sunlight for 24 hours. Some of the common photosensitizing essential oils include:

ANGELICA ROOT
BERGAMOT
CUMIN
DISTILLED OR EXPRESSED GRAPEFRUIT
EXPRESSED LEMON
EXPRESSED LIME
ORANGE, BITTER
RUE

This is also a partial list, so exercise caution and good judgment when applying an essential oil.

CAUTION: HUMANS AND PETS RESPOND TO ESSENTIAL OILS DIFFERENTLY

Do not assume that what is good for you will be the equivalent (or even safe) for an animal. It is best to consult first with a veterinarian and a trained aromatherapist before administering *any* essential oil for your pet's health.

Essential oils have sometimes been used for dogs, horses, and some other farm animals. In these cases they have been used topically for spot application and hoof/paw care. Inhalation therapy has also been used.

As a general rule, do not use *any* essential oil topically on cats. Their metabolic systems do not break down many of the substances contained in essential oils. Liver or kidney damage, or worse, may result when cats are exposed to essential oils. This can even include

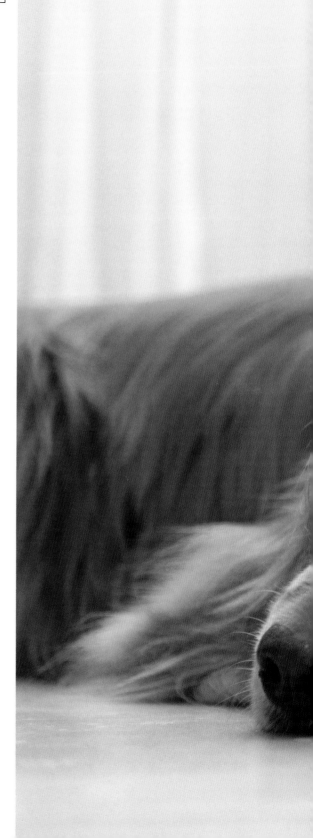

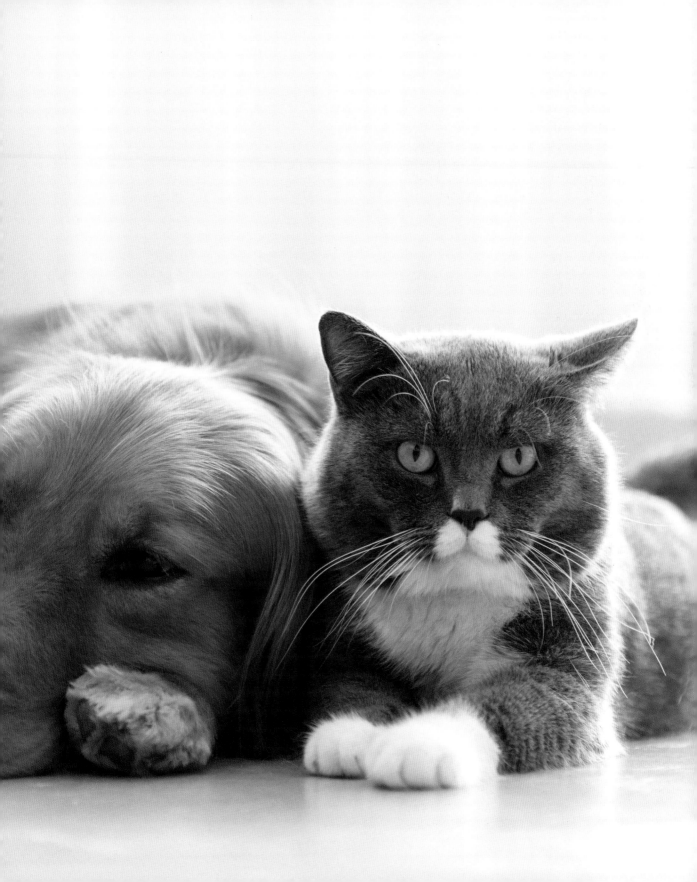

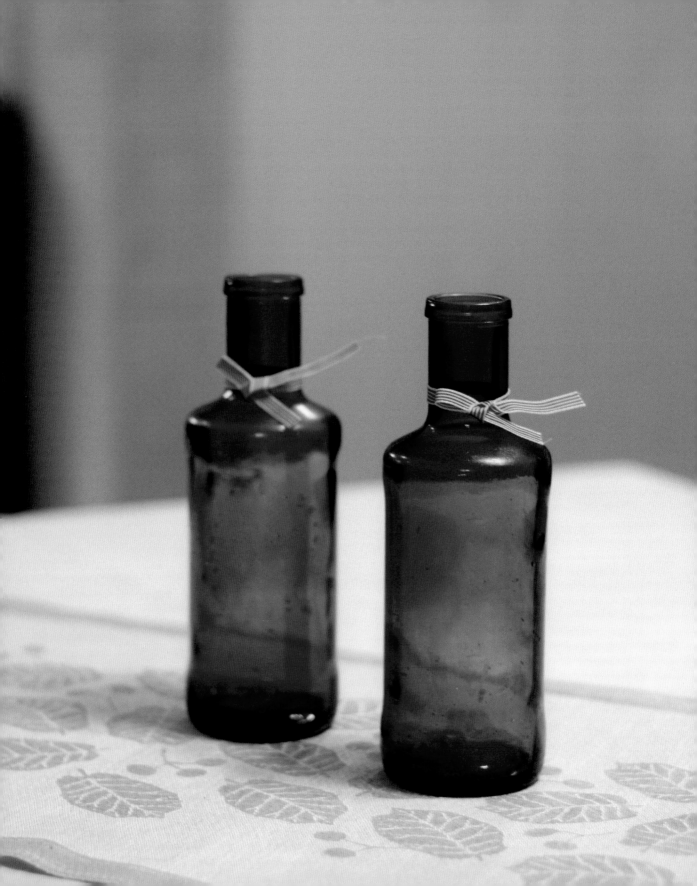

exposure to essential oils via diffusion. You should use the same extreme caution with fish, reptiles, birds, rodents, and small mammals.

STORAGE

Once you've purchased quality essential oils, you certainly will want to keep them that way. Store them in glass containers. Some essential oils can actually dissolve plastic, and storing them even temporarily in plastic may contaminate the oil. Don't store your essential oils in dropper bottles either, as it doesn't take long for the rubber seals and squeeze bulbs to melt into a gooey mess.

Be sure to keep essential oils out of direct sunlight and away from heat so they don't lose their potency. Keep them in a dark cupboard or medicine cabinet—not in a car or on a window ledge or sitting out in a bright room. Dark, amber-colored, cobalt blue, and green bottles are fairly common and are reasonably priced. They will protect your oils from the occasional damaging ultraviolet light. Make sure your caps are airtight.

If you have purchased a large bottle of essential oil, it's a good idea to transfer its contents to a smaller bottle once the bottle is half empty. This will help avoid oxidation. Remember: the less empty space in a bottle, the better.

Essential oils are natural preservatives and will help preserve your carrier oils. Their scent will change and fade over time,

however, and eventually lose quality. Properly stored, most oils will keep for at least several years. The citrus oils, such as orange and lemon, are most vulnerable to losing their smell, but even they will keep for a couple of years if refrigerated.

A few essential oils, including patchouli, clary sage, benzoin, vetiver, and sandalwood, actually help fix the scent of other aromas combined with them. And they get better with age. The same is true for thick resins such as myrrh. Patchouli that has been stored for many years smells so rich, few people recognize it—even those who otherwise dislike it! Essential oils such as these become yet more valuable with age.

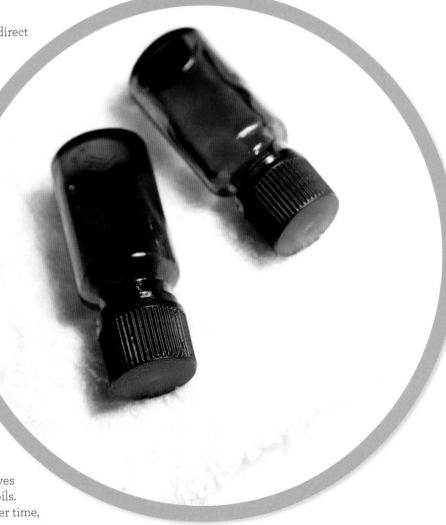

SUPPLIES

A measuring cup, measuring spoons, and perhaps some small funnels will start you on the road to aromatherapy production. Unless you are adding essential oils to a ready-made product, you will need appropriate bottles or containers for storage. Simple bottles and vials are sold at drugstores; for fancier ones, check out your local natural food store or essential oil retailers online. Buy some labels for the bottles, too. Make sure to have paper towels and rubbing alcohol on hand for cleanup.

You will need a way to measure small amounts of the essential oils and transfer them from bottle to bottle. Some essential oils are sold in bottles that have an insert called a reducer that allows only a drop of oil to come out at a time. It may take a few tries to get comfortable using it, but do not shake the bottle or several drops will come out at once. Glass droppers work well for obtaining just the right amount of essential oil. Be careful not to contaminate your essential oils by putting a dropper from one oil into another, but you don't need a separate dropper for each oil. Simply rinse the dropper in rubbing alcohol and wait a few minutes for the alcohol to completely evaporate before putting it into another oil. Having two or three droppers allows you to rotate them for rinsing and drying.

If you prefer, use a long, narrow tube called a pipette to measure out small amounts of essential oils. Pipettes can be made of glass or plastic; however, the easiest to use— but hardest to clean—is plastic with a squeeze bulb at one end. Practice

with these using water before attempting to get exact measurements with your essential oils. To measure larger quantities, use a Pyrex measuring cup with a pour spout. A set of measuring spoons is also useful for measuring more than a few drops of essential oil.

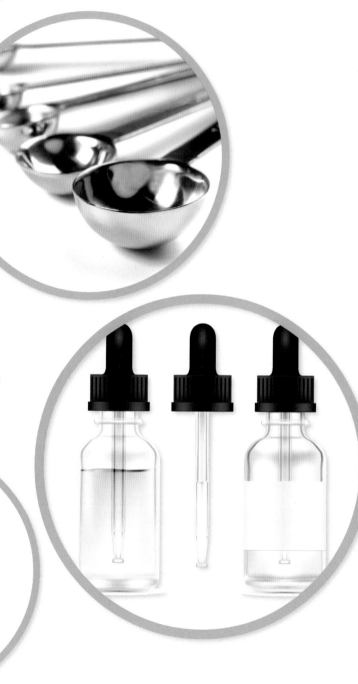

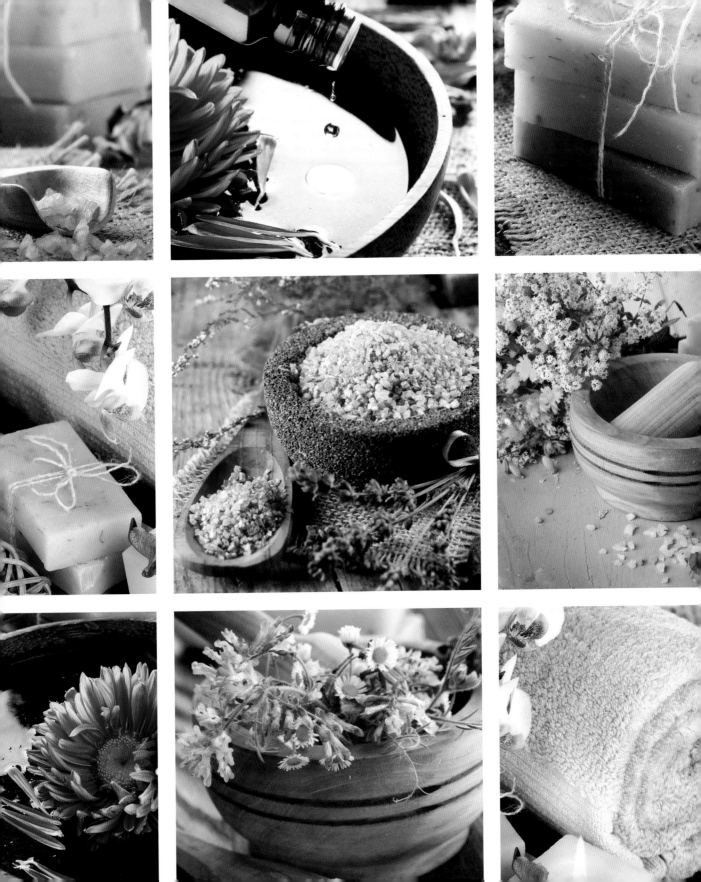

DILUTIONS

Some people find it easier to measure drops. Others prefer measuring essential oils by the teaspoon. It depends on how much you need to measure at one time and the width of the container into which it's going.

The size of a drop varies, depending on the size of the dropper opening and the temperature and viscosity (thickness) of the essential oil. Teaspoons are usually more convenient if you are preparing large quantities.

Most aromatherapy applications are a two-percent dilution. This means 2 drops of essential oil is added for every 100 drops of carrier oil—a safe and effective dilution for most aromatherapy applications. A one-percent dilution is suggested for children, pregnant women, and those who are weak from chronic illness. In some cases, you will want to use even less. Dilutions of three percent or more are used only for strong preparations such as liniments or for "spot" therapy, when you are only treating a tiny area instead of the entire body. Always remember that in aromatherapy, more is not necessarily better. In fact, too great a concentration may produce unwanted reactions. The following are standard dilutions:

• 1 percent dilution: 5–6 drops per ounce of carrier
• 2 percent dilution: 10–12 drops (about 1/8 teaspoon) per ounce of carrier
• 3 percent dilution: 15–18 drops (a little less than 1/4 teaspoon) per ounce of carrier

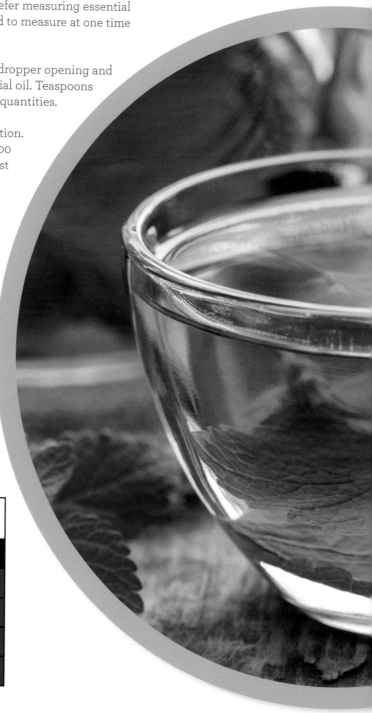

MEASUREMENT CONVERSIONS

drops	tsp	oz	dram	ml
12.5	1/8	1/48	1/6	5/8
25	1/4	1/24	1/3	1 1/4
75	3/4	1/8	1	3.7
100	1	1/6	1 1/3	5

BLENDING

For your very first aromatherapy blends, keep it simple. Use your favorite essential oils, but preferably no more than three to five at a time. Later, the many choices of oils will add to the excitement of creating your own blends.

Keep an aromatherapy notebook from the very beginning—you'll need exact records of how you made all your preparations. Jot down the ingredients, proportions, and processing procedures you used for each blend, as well as observations about how well it worked. Label your finished products with the ingredients, date, and special instructions, if any. You will be thankful for this information later when you come up with a formula everyone loves, and you want to duplicate it.

When considering new blends, try to think first about the characteristics of each oil, including what professional perfumers call personality, aroma notes, and odor intensity. Perfumers think of each oil as having its own unique personality, and they think of scent

in terms of a musical scale: Fragrances have head or top notes, middle or heart notes, and base notes. The top notes are the odors that are smelled first but evaporate quickly, the heart is the scent that emerges after the first fifteen minutes, while the base note is the scent that lingers hours later.

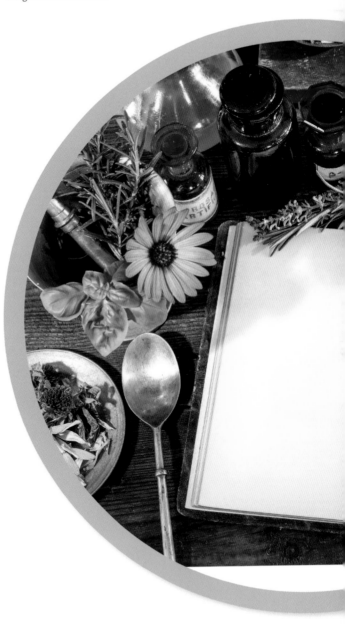

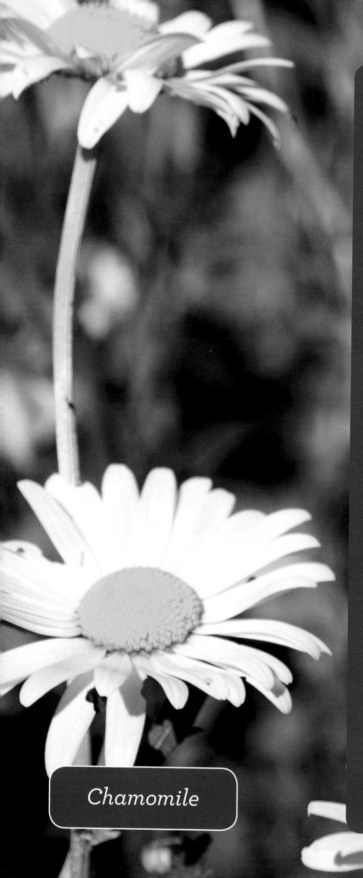

Chamomile

BASIC ESSENTIAL OIL STARTER KIT

Lavender—fights inflammation, infection, insomnia, pain, depression, anxiety; appropriate for all complexion and hair types.

Chamomile—aids digestion, promotes relaxation, treats allergies, menstrual cramps, depression, inflammation, anxiety, anger, rashes, and dry and problem skin, complexion, and hair.

Rosemary—relieves pain, congestion, constipation and grief; stimulates circulation and memory; appropriate for most complexion and hair types.

Tea tree—fights most types of infection; appropriate for oily skin and hair.

Peppermint—relieves indigestion, sinus congestion, itching, and panic; mental stimulant; use small amounts for dry skin and hair.

Lemon, orange, or other citrus—antidepressant; kills parasites; appropriate for oily complexion and hair.

Geranium—excellent mind/body balancer; appropriate for all complexion and hair types.

COMPRESS

An aromatherapy compress concentrates essential oils in a specific area of the body and keeps the area moist. It is one of the quickest and easiest therapeutic techniques to make. Add about 5 drops of an essential oil or a blend of oils to a cup of water. Use hot or cold water, whichever is best for the particular treatment: Cold water helps relieve itching, swelling, and inflammation, while hot water increases circulation and opens pores, helping to flush out blemishes. Fold a soft cloth and soak it in the water; then wring it out and apply it where needed. If you feel overheated, try a cold compress on your forehead. Cold is also usually the preferred temperature for relieving strained eyes. A cool compress can also help to get rid of a headache, although a few people find that heat works better for them. A hot compress against the back of the neck will relieve neck strain and tight muscles.

FOOT OR HAND BATH

Soaking your hands or feet in an aromatherapy mini-bath is an excellent treatment for stiffness, aches, and skin irritations. In fact, your entire body will benefit since the essential oils penetrate the skin and enter the bloodstream. To make a foot or hand bath, simply add 5 to 10 drops of essential oil to a quart of hot or cold water in a large basin. Stir well to distribute the essential oils, then soak your feet or hands for at least five minutes. Cold water reduces swelling while warm water relaxes stiff muscles. To improve leg circulation in conditions such as varicose veins, alternate between a hot and cold bath.

INHALANT

Steam inhalations are a great way to treat any upper respiratory or sinus problem. The steam carries essential oils directly to sinuses and lungs, where they fight infection. Additionally, the warm, moist air opens nasal and bronchial passages, making it easier to breathe. To create a steam inhalant, bring about 3 cups of water to a boil in a pan. Turn off the heat, and add 3–5 drops of essential oil to the water. Drape a towel over both your head and the pan to capture the steam, keeping your eyes closed and your head about 12 inches from the water. Take deep, relaxing breaths of the fragrant steam. You can also humidify and disinfect an entire room—just keep the mixture on a very low simmer. Essential oils can also be used in many humidifiers.

When you're away from home and steam inhalation treatments are impractical, inhale a tissue scented with the oils or use a natural nasal inhaler, which can be found at natural food stores.

LINIMENT

Liniments increase circulation. Rub them externally on the skin to warm muscles and to reduce muscle and joint pain. Liniments also disinfect wounds and dry up skin eruptions. Fitness experts suggest applying liniment before exercising, not afterwards, so that it can work like a mini-warm-up, heating muscles so they will stretch better. (Don't use this as an excuse to skimp on your stretches, however!) Make a quick and easy liniment by adding 15–20 drops of the appropriate heating essential oils, such as peppermint and clove, for every ounce of alcohol, oil, or vinegar. Alcohol is cooling and quickly evaporates, leaving no oily residue. Oil heats up faster and stays on the skin longer, making it more like a concentrated massage.

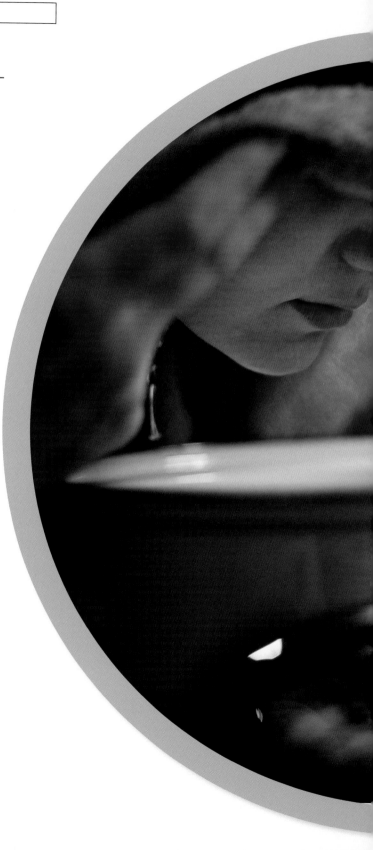

SALVE

Salves are made of herbal oils that are thickened with beeswax, so they form a healing and protective coating that adheres better to the skin. They are used on almost all skin problems, such as minor cuts, bruises, scrapes, diaper or heat rash, insect bites, eczema, psoriasis, and swelling. You can make any salve aromatherapeutic by stirring 24 drops of essential oil into 2 ounces of salve. This is fairly easy to do with a toothpick. The resulting salve will be a little runnier than usual, but it will stick to the skin perfectly well.

SITZ BATH

A "sitz" bath is simply a mini-bath that employs hot and cold water to increase blood circulation, primarily in the pelvic region. This makes it ideal for uterine or bladder problems. Add 5–10 drops of essential oil to a bathtub containing about 10 inches of water (up to your waist). The water temperature should be as hot as you can easily stand but not so hot as to hurt. Prepare a small tub of cold water and leave it nearby. Sit in the hot water 5 to 10 minutes. Quickly remove yourself to the tub of cold water and sit in it for at least 1 minute. The large plastic tubs sold at hardware stores are well-suited for this purpose. Continue alternating between the hot and cold tubs for a total of two to five times each. Repeat the treatment every day for 3 to 5 days.

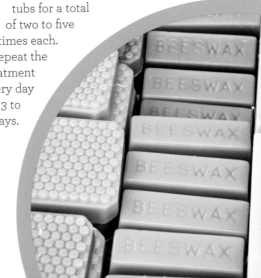

BATH SALTS

1 teaspoon essential oil (your choice)
1 cup borax
1/2 cup sea salt
1/2 cup baking soda

Mix salts together, and add essential oils, mixing well to combine. Use 1/4 to 1/2 cup of the bath salts per bath. For muscle aches and pains, add 1/2 cup Epsom salts to this recipe. (All of these salts are sold in grocery stores.) This makes a very relaxing and soothing bath. Sea salt softens water and makes more soap suds, so you can use much less soap. This is good because soap can be harsh on delicate skin. This mix also makes the skin feel smooth, although in excess, it may be drying to already dry skin.

AROMATIC WATERS

Scented waters treat many different skin problems, such as acne and burns, and are also used cosmetically as a skin-freshener. The essential oils they contain are so diluted that aromatic waters can be applied directly onto sensitive areas of the face. They are perfect for making herbal compresses for injured skin or for complexion problems. Although different from hydrosols, which are the more expensive by-products of distilling essential oils, these aromatic waters work wonderfully in their own right. Add 5–10 drops of fragrant essential oils to 4 ounces of water or aloe vera juice.

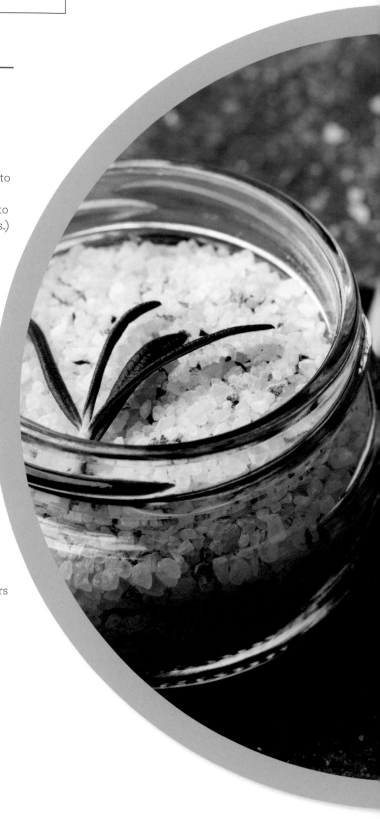

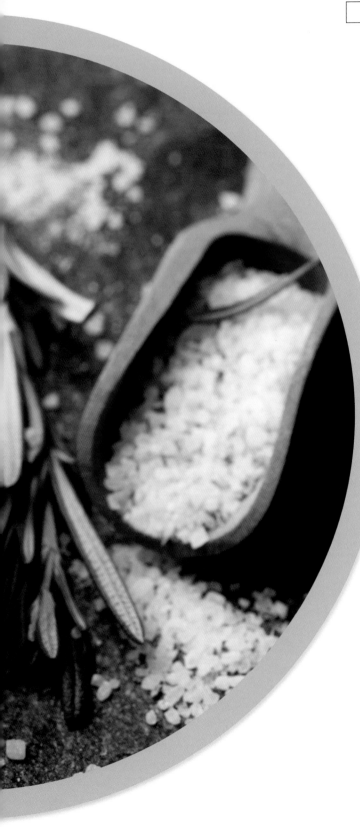

CREAM

1 cup oil
3/4 ounce beeswax (22 grams), shaved
1 cup distilled water, warm
30 to 50 drops essential oils

Making cream is very similar to making mayonnaise—the proportions need to be fairly exact for it to come out right. Carefully melt the shaved beeswax in the oil on the stove. Cool it so that you can put your finger in the oil without discomfort. Put the lid on your blender with the center cap removed. Pour the warm water into the blender through a funnel (using a wide mouth funnel reduces splattering). Turn the blender on high speed, and add the oil/beeswax mixture slowly and evenly. It should begin to thicken after about three fourths of the oil has been added. This is a good time to add the essential oils. When all of the oil has been added, you will have a thick, beautiful cream. Pour the cream into wide-mouth jars. The cream will last at least a month if kept in a cool place. Storing it in the refrigerator will prolong its shelf life for several months.

DEODORANT

The most important action of any deodorant is to kill bacteria, which essential oils do very well. By making your own deodorant, you can soothe rashes and irritations (try Roman chamomile) and avoid the use of the harsh, pore-blocking ingredients found in commercial products.

15 drops lavender oil
5 drops sage oil
5 drops coriander oil
2 ounces aloe vera juice or witch hazel

Combine all ingredients in a spray bottle. Shake well before each use. This will keep at least a year.

POTPOURRI

Few things grace a room more than an attractive container of dried flowers, herbs, woods, and spices, freshening a room with its gentle and perhaps seasonal background aroma. Modern potpourris owe most of their fragrance to essential oils added to dried herbs. The basic recipe is 1/2 teaspoon essential oil to 2 cups dried herbs.

Since some essential oils have the unique property of becoming better with age, these can be used as fixatives. They will preserve the fragrance, making it last long after it would otherwise dissipate. The potpourri also smells better with the addition of such oils as patchouli, sandalwood, benzoin, clary sage, balsam of Peru, balsam of tolu, vetiver, and orris root, used either as the chopped herb or in the form of an essential oil. The most popular potpourri fixative is orris root. It has a light, violet-like fragrance that blends with any scent, and it is not over-powering. Although a few people are allergic to orris, it is still the all-time favorite. Its essential oil is so rare that orris is added in its chopped form.

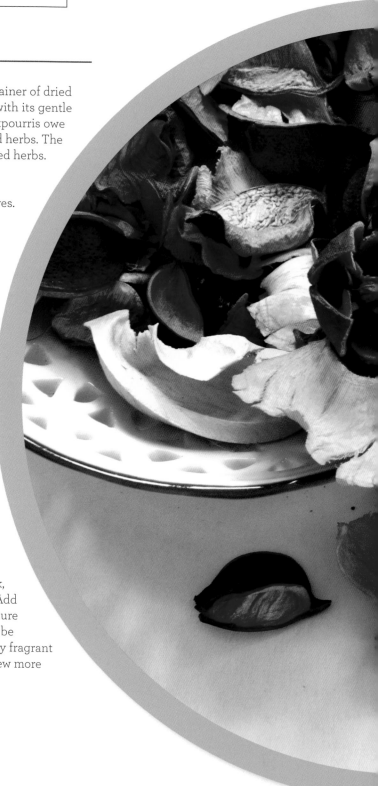

POTPOURRI BASE

1 cup mixed herbs, dried
1 tablespoon orris root, chopped
1/4 teaspoon essential oil
(twice the amount for simmering potpourri)

Use any combination of attractive flowers, leaves, bark, wood shavings, or cones for the dried plant material. Add the orris root and essential oils and stir. Keep the mixture in a closed container for several days so the scent can be absorbed by the plant material. This potpourri will stay fragrant for many months. When it gets faint, revive it with a few more drops of essential oil.

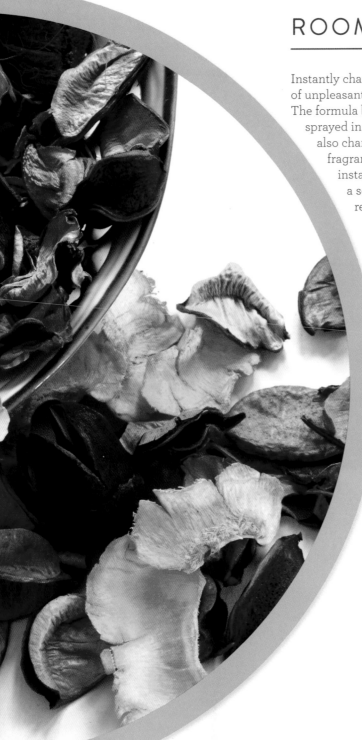

ROOM SPRAY

Instantly change the energy in a room, cleanse the air, or get rid of unpleasant odors by using an aromatherapeutic room spray. The formula below is a multipurpose room disinfectant. It can be sprayed in a sick room or used on the kitchen counter. You can also change the oils to create a spray that will make the room fragrant or that will impact the emotions. One mom, for instance, sprays her children's bedrooms every evening with a soothing chamomile and ylang ylang mix that helps relax them for sleep.

DISINFECTANT ROOM SPRAY

4 drops eucalyptus (or tea tree) oil
3 drops lavender oil
2 drops bergamot oil
2 drops thyme oil
1 drop peppermint oil
2 ounces water

Add the essential oils to the water. Keep in a spritzer bottle (sold in most drug stores and some cosmetic stores). Be sure to shake the bottle very well right before using to help distribute the essential oils in the water. Otherwise, they tend to float on the surface.

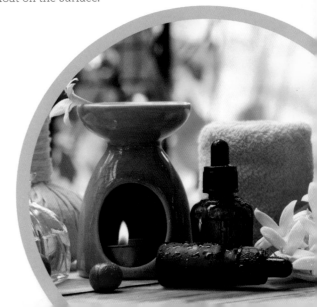

MOTH-PROOF SACHET

Sachets freshen clothing and keep moths and other insects away.

20 drops cedarwood
8 drops lavender
8 drops patchouli or sage
1 dozen cotton balls

Combine essential oils and place about 3 drops on each cotton ball. Store in a closed container for a couple days. Place with clothes, using them instead of commercial moth balls (about six for an average sized box or suitcase). To make more attractive balls, tie a small fabric square around the cotton ball.

SCENTED CANDLE

Impregnated with essential oils, candles release the scent as they burn, creating whatever mood you want. You can make an aromatherapy candle from a purchased unscented candle by adding several drops of essential oil to the candle's wick. Wait 24 hours, until the wick absorbs the oil, before using the candle. You can make scented candles from scratch by adding oil to the melted wax or by saturating the wick just before pouring the candle. The wick method uses less oil, but many people like the scent of the candle.

CITRONELLA CANDLE

1 votive candle
20 drops citronella

Using a glass dropper, drop the oil on the candle's wick. Wait 24 hours before using.

VACUUM CLEANER

Drop 2 to 4 drops of oil directly into the bag. Not only does the oil disinfect the dirt, but it will brighten your day. Try lemon eucalyptus—it is highly antiseptic, and the lemon gives people a feeling of cleanliness. In addition, its stimulating properties will help you get that housework done!

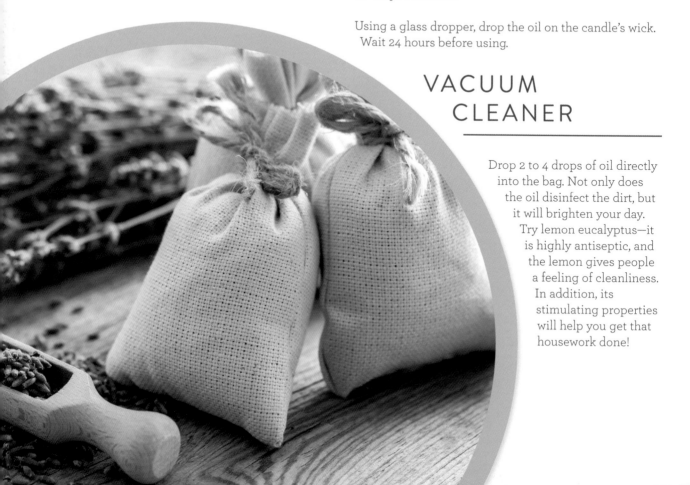

ALLSPICE

BOTANICAL NAME: *PIMENTA DIOICA*

Contrary to popular belief, allspice is not simply a mixture of "all spices." However, the dried fruit of the *pimenta dioica* plant—an evergreen native to the Caribbean and South America—does have a unique aroma reminiscent of several different spices. The name was coined sometime in the early 17th century, thanks to its notes of cinnamon, clove, cardamom, nutmeg, and pepper. This versatile ingredient is a staple in Caribbean and Middle Eastern cuisine, and can often be found in seasonal desserts in the U.S. But the plant's benefits go beyond food: the essential oil is prized for many health and beauty uses.

THERAPEUTIC PROPERTIES

Antioxidant and antiseptic; analgesic; aids digestion; used in perfumes, candles, and cosmetics.

USED FOR

Allspice oil contains antioxidant compounds including methyl eugenol and cineol, as well as vitamins A, B, and C. This makes it excellent for fighting oxidative stress in the body. The oil can be used to treat wounds and prevent infections. When rubbed into joints and muscles, its analgesic effects provide soothing relief for arthritis, muscle strains, and insect bites. Allspice is known for its ability to ease diarrhea, indigestion, and vomiting. And a few drops mixed with sugar and coconut oil create an aromatic face scrub.

PRECAUTIONS

Allspice should always be used with a carrier oil, as it can be irritating to the skin when undiluted.

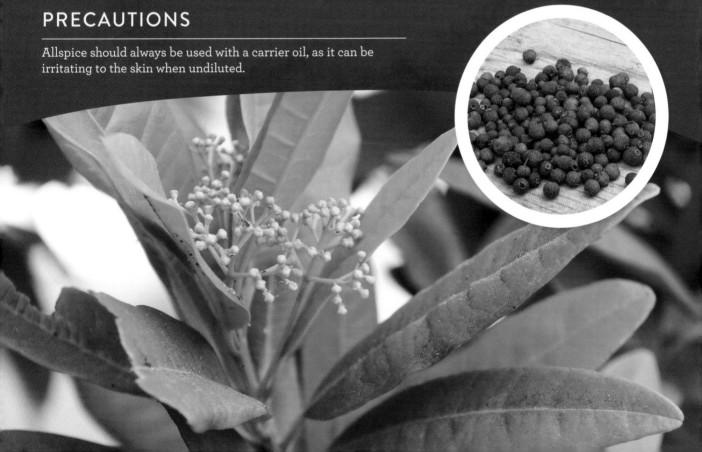

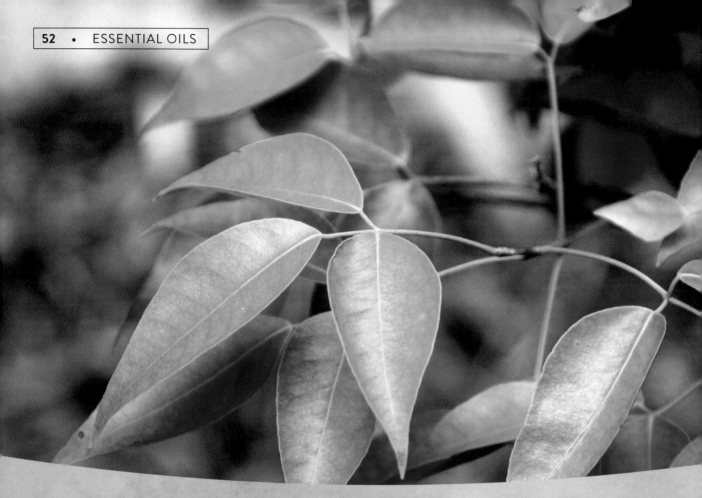

AMYRIS

BOTANICAL NAME: *AMYRIS BALSAMIFERA*

The amyris is an evergreen tree found in the wild mostly in Haiti and the Dominican Republic. The leaves and white flowers of the tree smell citrusy when they are crushed, and, in fact, the tree derived its name from the Greek word *amyron*, which means "intensely scented." Amyris is often also known as torchwood or candlewood, because the prized oil within the wood is highly combustible. Branches can be used for torches or candles, all the while emitting a pleasant scent. The oil itself has a woody, sweet fragrance, and is extracted from the wood by steam distillation.

THERAPEUTIC PROPERTIES

Antiseptic, anti-inflammatory, sedative, decongestant, and emollient properties; the scent works well for aromatherapy.

USED FOR

Amyris oil is often used in soaps and perfumes because of its scent, but its antimicrobial properties make it effective on acne, rashes, dry skin, and minor cuts and scrapes. It can also be used to calm upset stomachs and aid in digestion. It works well in a diffuser or as incense to create a peaceful, relaxing atmosphere.

ANGELICA ROOT

BOTANICAL NAME: *ANGELICA ARCHANGELICA*

Commonly known as garden angelica, wild celery, or Norwegian angelica, angelica comes from the same plant family as carrots, parsnips, and fennel. The biennial plant—native to northern Europe and Greenland—is grown for its edible stems and sweet-smelling roots, which have been used medicinally since the 10th century. Its healing properties are so prized that the oil is also known as Holy Spirit Root, Archangel Root, and the Oil of Angels. Additionally, there are around 80 different aroma compounds found in angelica root, giving the essential oil its distinctive smell of musk and making it a favorite of perfumers and the food and beverage industry.

THERAPEUTIC PROPERTIES

Antispasmodic; aids digestion; helps relieve stress and anxiety.

USED FOR

Angelica root's antispasmodic properties make it useful for relieving cramps, coughs, and muscle aches. It has been shown to be useful for treating gastritis, stomach ulcers, gas, and indigestion. Angelica root has a lovely fragrance on its own, and it also blends well with other essential oils; this makes it excellent for use in calming aromatherapy.

PRECAUTIONS

Sun exposure should be avoided for 12 hours after using angelica root oil to avoid phototoxicity. The oil should not be used by diabetics or pregnant women.

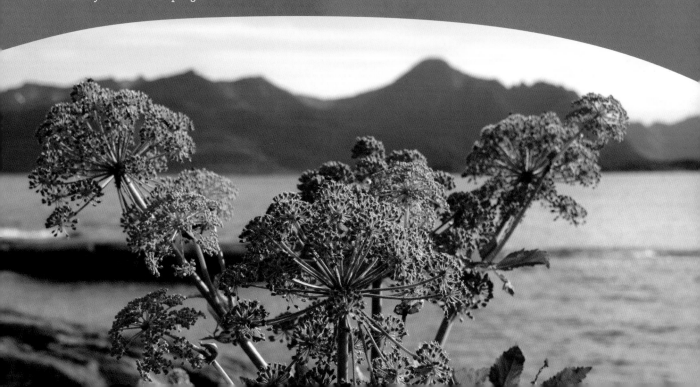

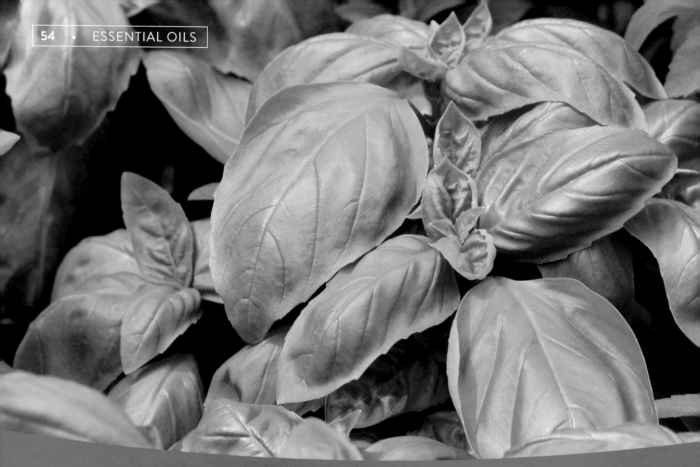

BASIL

BOTANICAL NAME: *OCIMUM BASILICUM*

Named after the Greek *basileus*, meaning "king," basil—the "king of herbs"—has been cultivated in India for at least 5,000 years. It has been used for culinary purposes in Asian and Mediterranean cultures for centuries, and today many of us know it mostly as an essential pizza and pesto ingredient. But the tasty herb was often used in ancient Chinese and Ayurvedic medicinal practices to treat coughs, fevers, indigestion, constipation, and skin rashes. The herb is also used in religious practices in the Eastern Orthodox Church and Hinduism. The spicy, herby scented oil can be diluted in olive or coconut oil and applied topically, or used in a diffuser.

THERAPEUTIC PROPERTIES

Aids digestion; has antibacterial, antiviral, and analgesic properties; muscle relaxant; repels some insects.

USED FOR

Research has shown that basil oil is effective at fighting bacteria and fungi, making it an excellent choice for a natural kitchen and bathroom cleaner. The oil also helps to kill odor-causing bacteria and mold on furniture, kitchen appliances, or in your car. You can use the oil when fighting colds or the flu by diffusing it in your home, or adding a few drops to a bath. Try adding a few drops of basil oil to coconut oil and rubbing into sore, painful muscles. The oil can also be used to make bug repellent, mouthwash, or toothpaste.

BAY (LAUREL)

BOTANICAL NAME: *LAURUS NOBILIS*

The leaves of the bay laurel plant are probably best known for their use as a flavoring agent in soups and stocks. They also became a symbol of wealth and victory in ancient Greece and Rome, where laurel wreaths were worn as fashion or given as prizes. Traditionally, the plant was used medicinally to alleviate stomach ailments, and the essential oil has been used to create the famous "Aleppo soap" since antiquity. Today, the ornamental plant is still popular in the Mediterranean region, and the essential oil distilled from its aromatic leaves is prized for its many health benefits and spicy scent.

THERAPEUTIC PROPERTIES

Antiseptic, antibacterial; analgesic; helps to relieve symptoms of colds and flu; aids digestion; can be used as an insecticide.

USED FOR

Use bay oil to treat minor cuts and scrapes. Its analgesic properties make it an excellent choice for relieving aches and pains, especially achy muscles due to colds and flu. Used in aromatherapy, bay oil also helps calm coughs and ease congestion. It has been used to ease digestive upset for centuries. The strong scent of the oil can help to repel insects.

PRECAUTIONS

Can cause skin irritation, and should always be diluted in a carrier oil before using.

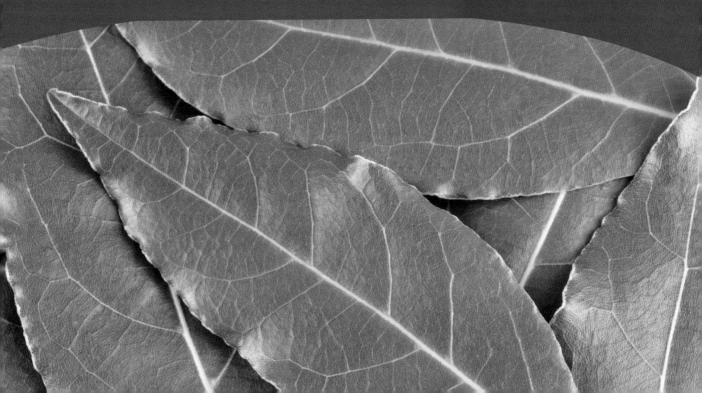

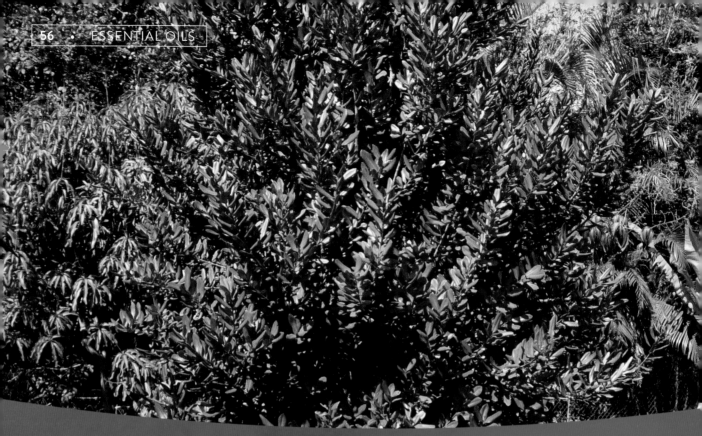

(WEST INDIAN) BAY

BOTANICAL NAME: *PIMENTA RACEMOSA*

Often confused with bay laurel oil, West Indian bay oil is derived from a different plant. "The spice tree," as it's sometimes called in its native Caribbean, is an evergreen tree with highly aromatic leaves. Also called sweet bay and bay rum, the tree produces leaves with a unique scent: a combination of cinnamon, clove, nutmeg, vanilla, and cardamom. The leaves are prized in traditional Caribbean cooking and are used in the West Indies for making tea, as an air freshener, and as bug repellent. In the early 20th century, the essential oil was used to create bay rum cologne, a scent that is still popular in men's toiletry products.

THERAPEUTIC PROPERTIES

Antimicrobial; analgesic; insecticide; frequently used as a fragrance.

USED FOR

Bay oil's antimicrobial properties and spicy scent make it a popular treatment for scalp conditions like dandruff and flaky scalp. When used as a massage oil, it can help relieve aches and pains. The oil can be used to repel insects, and is particularly helpful in warding off moths. The classic scent of bay rum is found in many colognes, soaps, aftershaves, and deodorants.

PRECAUTIONS

Antimicrobial; analgesic; insecticide; frequently used as a fragrance.

BENZOIN

BOTANICAL NAME: *STYRAX BENZOIN*

The trunk of the benzoin tree exudes a vanilla-scented gum resin when cut. Used since antiquity in medicine, it was imported by the Arabs to use as a less expensive substitute for frankincense. They made pomades that smelled like vanilla and were rubbed on the skin for fragrance and healing. Traders brought benzoin to Greece, Rome, and Egypt, where it became prized as a fixative in perfumes—still one of its uses today. Europeans highly regarded benzoin for its medicinal properties as well as its scent. Benzoin is typically sold as an absolute, but it is so thick it may be difficult for you to get it out of the bottle. If so, dilute it with a little alcohol or dissolve it in warm carrier oil so it is easier to pour.

THERAPEUTIC PROPERTIES

Antibacterial, antifungal, antioxidant; seals wounds from infection; counteracts inflammation; decreases gas, indigestion, and lung congestion; promotes circulation.

USED FOR

Effective against redness, irritation, or itching on the skin, benzoin's most popular use is in a cream to protect chapped skin and improve skin elasticity. Since it is also a strong preservative, adding it to vegetable oil–based preparations delays their oxidation and spoilage. Benzoin essential oil can be added to chest rub balms and massage oils for lung and sinus ailments.

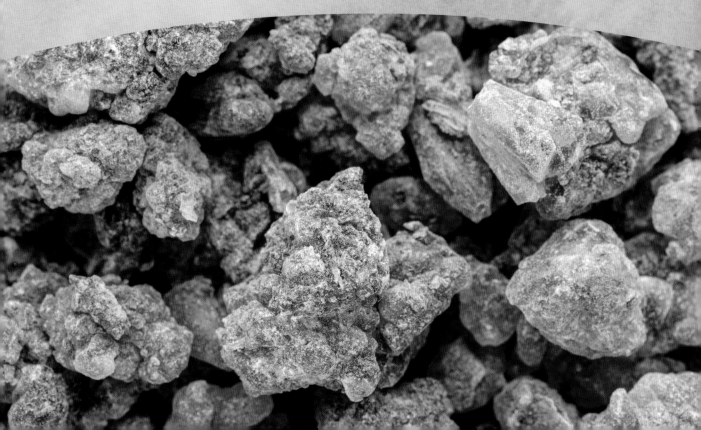

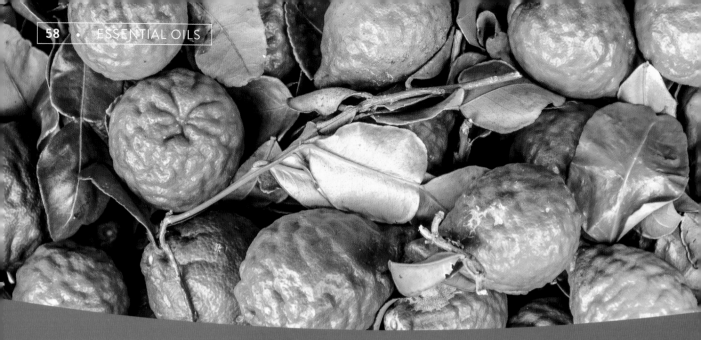

BERGAMOT

BOTANICAL NAME: *CITRUS BERGAMIA*

A small citrus tree originally from tropical Asia, it produces the round, green fruit whose oils are expressed from the rinds before ripening. While not edible or pretty, they smell truly wonderful! The green-tinted oil gained favor only after the tree was brought to Bergamot, Italy, in the fifteenth century. There it was used to treat fevers, malaria, and intestinal worms. According to legend, Christopher Columbus brought the tree to the Caribbean, where it was popularly used in voodoo practices to protect one from misfortune. Modern aromatherapists suggest placing a few drops of bergamot on a cloth and carrying it in your pocket or travel bag. Sniff the scented cloth while traveling to reduce stress, depression, anxiety, or insomnia.

THERAPEUTIC PROPERTIES

Antiseptic, anti-inflammatory, antidepressant, antiviral, antibiotic.

USED FOR

Bergamot fights several viruses, including those that cause flu, herpes, shingles, and chicken pox. Due to its versatile antibiotic properties, it also treats bacterial infections of the urinary system, mouth, and throat. It is helpful for a variety of skin conditions, including eczema. The best way to use it is diluted in a salve or massage oil that is applied externally over the afflicted area. As a natural deodorant, it not only provides a pleasant scent, but it kills bacteria that are responsible for odor.

PRECAUTIONS

Due to bergapten, bergamot can cause abnormal skin pigmentation when used externally by sensitive individuals who then go out in the sun. A bergapten-free essential oil is available; this should be noted on the bottle. While it may sound appealing to make your own Earl Grey tea, leave that up to the experts; they add only the tiniest amount of essential oil in a quantity that is safe to ingest.

BIRCH

BOTANICAL NAME: *BETULA LENTA*

The scent and flavor of birch has been a European and North American Indian favorite for centuries. Birch drinks were favored by those suffering from consumption because the natural aspirin, methyl salicylate, in the essential oil relieves pain and makes it easier to breathe.

THERAPEUTIC PROPERTIES

Astringent, antiseptic; promotes menstruation; alleviates joint pain.

USED FOR

In a massage oil or liniment, birch can be rubbed over painful areas to ease muscular and arthritic pain and stiffness. Alternatively, a couple drops of birch essential oil, along with a drop or two of another oil such as lavender to soften birch's sharp scent, can be added to your bath for the same purpose. This type of aromatherapy bath is also useful to increase circulation and promote menstruation, especially when delayed by physical or emotional stress. A salve or lotion containing birch essential oil softens the roughness caused by psoriasis, eczema, and other skin problems.

PRECAUTIONS

Be sure not to overdo the suggested quantities of this potent essential oil, as it can be toxic in high doses. Since it smells like candy, store it safely away from children so they won't be tempted to taste it.

BLACK PEPPER

BOTANICAL NAME: *PIPER NIGRUM*

Traded more than any other spice in the world, black pepper has been prized since antiquity not only for its flavor-enhancing spiciness, but also for its medicinal usefulness. The spice has been found in ancient Egyptian tombs, was frequently used in ancient Roman cookery, and was so coveted by Europeans that it was briefly used as a form of currency. In fact, Alaric the Visigoth, famous for sacking the city of Rome in the year 410, demanded 3,000 pounds of pepper as a ransom for the city! The spice is obtained by cooking and drying the unripe fruit of the flowering vine. Once dried, oil can be extracted from the fruit by crushing it.

THERAPEUTIC PROPERTIES

Supports cell function, immune system, and circulation; antioxidant; provides a warming sensation when applied topically.

USED FOR

The warming properties of black pepper oil make it ideal for soothing sore muscles and aiding in relief from arthritis and rheumatism. A couple diluted drops rubbed into the affected area can help improve pain and ease mobility. Taken internally (again, diluted), black pepper oil protects the body from free radicals and helps to repair cell damage, and has even been shown to lower cholesterol. It may also aid digestion, and help to kill harmful bacteria in the body.

PRECAUTIONS

Black pepper oil should not be taken in large quantities, as it can cause vomiting, sleeplessness, and overheating. Also, care should be used when applying topically, as the warming sensation of the oil may be irritating for sensitive skin.

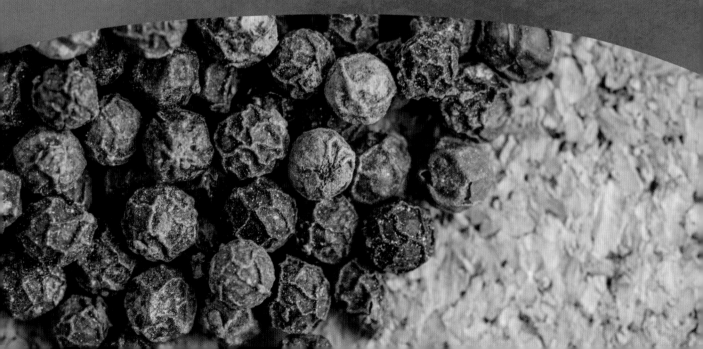

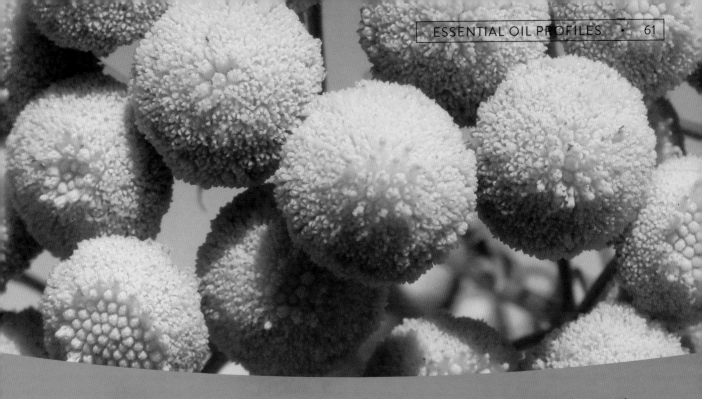

BLUE TANSY

BOTANICAL NAME: *TANACETUM ANNUUM*

True to its name, blue tansy essential oil is a unique, vibrant shade of cobalt, thanks to the presence of a compound called chamazulene. But interestingly, the flower from which the oil is derived is bright yellow. The flowering Mediterranean herb, native to Morocco, is similar to the common tansy with its lively-colored, button-like flowers. But the oil distilled from *Tanacetum annuum* is chemically different than the oil derived from its cousin, *Tanacetum vulgare*. Be sure to seek out a reputable seller, as occasionally a sneaky, unethical reseller will dilute blue tansy oil with the cheaper oil of the common tansy.

THERAPEUTIC PROPERTIES

Antibacterial, antifungal, and anti-inflammatory; analgesic; helps calm allergies.

USED FOR

Blue tansy oil helps prevent infections in cuts and scrapes, and its antibacterial and anti-inflammatory properties make it ideal for treating acne. A small amount added to shampoo can calm an itchy scalp. To relieve pain from arthritis or achy muscles, use blue tansy as a massage oil or add to a warm bath. Blue tansy is a natural antihistamine, and using in a steam inhaler can help quell sneezing, itchy eyes, or hives.

PRECAUTIONS

Because it has a high concentration of camphor, blue tansy should not be used by people with epilepsy or Parkinson's disease.

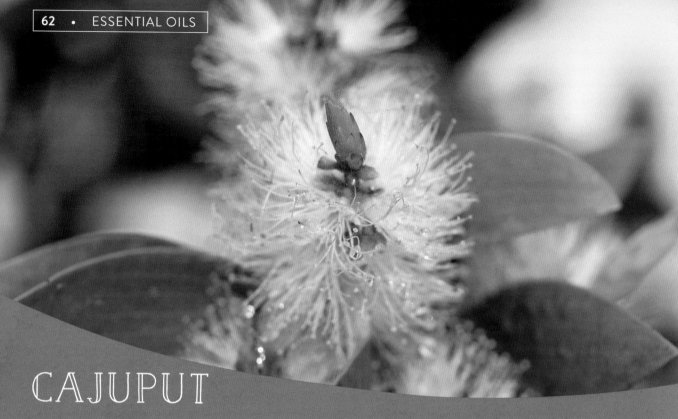

CAJUPUT

BOTANICAL NAME: *MELALEUCA CAJUPUTI*

Found mainly in Australia, Southeast Asia, and New Guinea, the cajuput tree has been used as a source of healing ingredients for centuries. Aboriginal Australians discovered that the leaves of the large, flowering tree could be used to treat aches and pains. They would also crush the leaves and inhale the vapors to ease respiratory ailments. And in Asia, the leaves were used to make comforting herbal teas and therapeutic liniments. Today, Cajuput essential oil is steam distilled from the leaves and twigs of the tree, and is often compared to tea tree oil. It has a pleasant warming property that is excellent for soothing sore muscles; but that's just one of this amazing oil's many benefits!

THERAPEUTIC PROPERTIES

Antibacterial, antifungal, and antiviral; decongestant; analgesic; insect repellent.

USED FOR

Cajuput is a great addition to a first aid kit due to its antiseptic properties. It can be applied to cuts and wounds to ward off bacterial, fungal, and viral infections, and can also be used to clear up acne or to treat skin conditions like psoriasis. Used in an inhaler, cajuput helps relieve congestion due to colds and flu. The oil's warming effects make it perfect for soothing achy, sore muscles, and it helps to improve circulation. Cajuput oil can be diluted in a carrier oil and rubbed on the skin to repel insects, or it can be sprayed around your home to keep out unwanted critters.

PRECAUTIONS

Those with asthma should avoid inhaling cajuput, as it can trigger an asthma attack. The oil should never be used with children.

CALAMUS

BOTANICAL NAME: *ACORUS CALAMUS*

Mentioned in the biblical book of Exodus as an ingredient in holy anointing oil, calamus—native to India and central Asia—has been prized since antiquity for its sweet, nutty, aromatic scent. By the late 16th century, it made its way to Britain, where it was often strewn across floors of homes and churches, producing a sweet scent as the leaves were crushed underfoot. Beyond its lovely smell, the plant, which is often known as "sweet flag," has many healing and therapeutic properties, and it has long been employed in Chinese and Ayurvedic medicine.

THERAPEUTIC PROPERTIES

Antibacterial; analgesic; excellent for use in aromatherapy; insect repellent.

USED FOR

Calamus oil can be used to fight infection in minor cuts and scrapes. A few drops in bath water help to improve circulation and relieve achy joints and muscles. Its sweet scent is said to be very calming and relaxing, and may even help to boost memory. Calamus makes an effective insect repellent, and is often used to prevent ticks from bothering cattle.

PRECAUTIONS

Calamus oil can be toxic if ingested, so it's best to consult with an expert before using. It should never be used by pregnant women.

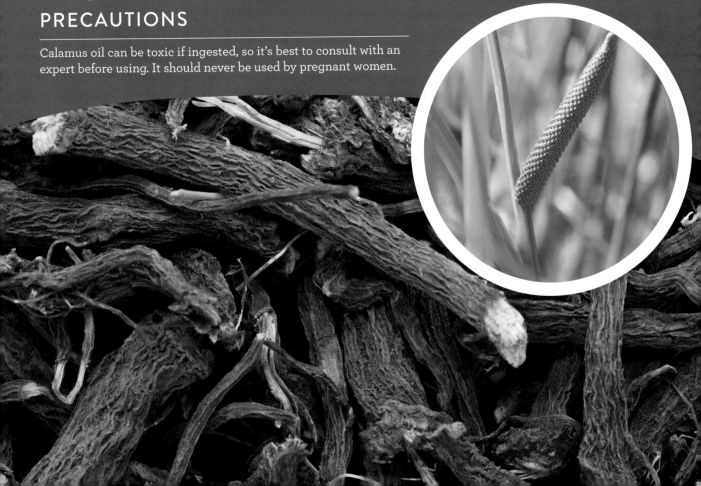

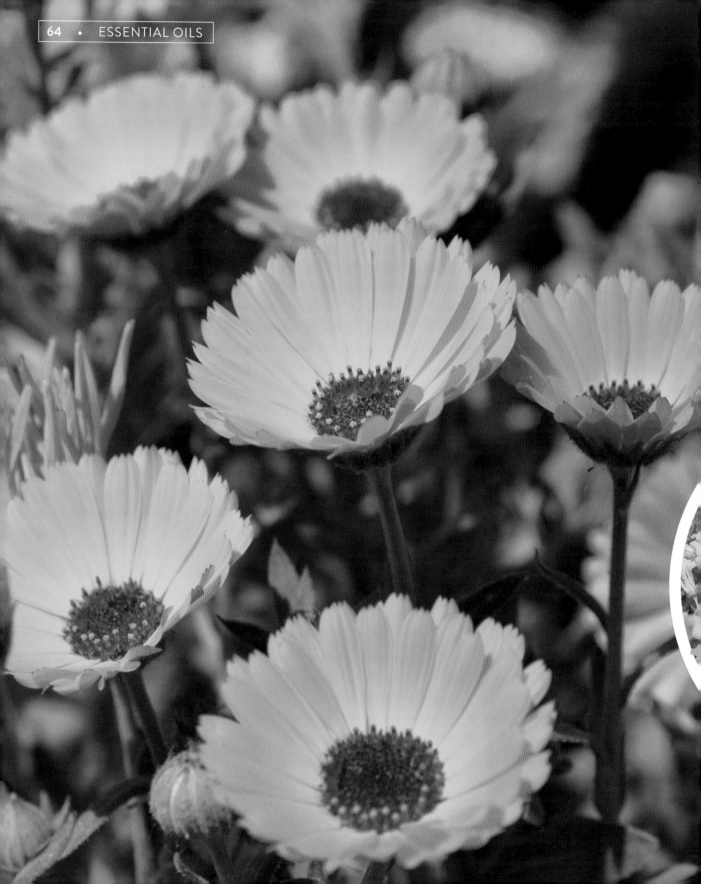

CALENDULA

BOTANICAL NAME: *CALENDULA OFFICINALIS*

Calendula—often referred to as the pot marigold—is an edible flower that has been used for centuries in European, Middle Eastern, and Mediterranean cooking. The bright yellow petals were sometimes used to add color to butter and cheese, or as a fabric dye. But calendula's usefulness goes far beyond its taste and color: the flower is mentioned in some of history's earliest medical texts, where it was recommended for aiding digestion, preventing infections, and detoxifying the liver. The flower was even used on the battlefield during the Civil War and World War I, as a remedy to prevent infection of open wounds. The sticky, syrupy oil distilled from the flowers is often extracted by steeping the petals in a hot carrier oil.

THERAPEUTIC PROPERTIES

Anti-inflammatory, antimicrobial, anti-viral; muscle relaxer; helps increase blood flow to injuries; improves skin firmness and hydration.

USED FOR

Calendula is a potent remedy for many inflammatory ailments, including dermatitis, ear infections, sore throats, ulcers, and diaper rash. Its muscle-relaxing properties can be used for abdominal cramps or constipation, and provide relief from PMS symptoms. It is also a popular additive in toothpastes, mouthwashes, and topical antiseptic ointments, due to its powerful antimicrobial properties.

PRECAUTIONS

Some people are allergic to calendula and other related plants, including ragweed, chamomile, and echinacea. Due to its muscle-relaxing properties, there is a possibility that it could interact negatively with some medications, including sedatives and diabetes or blood pressure medication. Pregnant women should also avoid calendula.

A LONG-VENERATED FLOWER

As a medicinal herb, calendula has been used in Europe since at least the 12th century. But even before that, it was revered by a number of civilizations. The name comes from the Latin *calends* (meaning the first day of the month), possibly because the Romans thought it would always bloom at this time. The ancient Greeks used it as a culinary garnish. The ancient Egyptians used the sap to heal wounds and help the skin regenerate. In fact, stylized calendula flowers appear in hieroglyphics that are thousands of years old.

Calendula is an unsurpassed skin healer. It assists in the healing of all manner of skin ailments, like cuts, abrasions, sunburn, bites, and bruises.

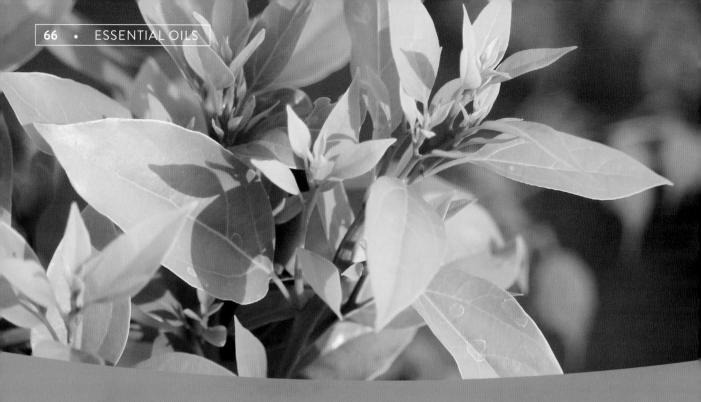

CAMPHOR

BOTANICAL NAME: *CINNAMOMUM CAMPHORA*

The camphor laurel is a large evergreen tree native to China, Japan, and other Asian countries. In fact, the third largest tree to ever grow in Japan is an 82-foot-tall camphor laurel, which is said to have first sprouted in prehistoric times! The wood and leaves of these trees are steam distilled to extract the essential oil, which has been used for centuries in everything from embalming fluid to medicines to insect repellent. Although researchers can't trace the first time the oil was ever used, they suspect that its strong scent and decongestant properties are what cemented camphor's place as a medicinal powerhouse.

THERAPEUTIC PROPERTIES

Decongestant, anesthetic, anti-inflammatory, disinfectant; insect repellent; stimulates circulatory system.

USED FOR

Camphor is popularly used as a decongestant because of its strong, sinus-clearing scent. It is also an excellent disinfectant, and can be added to ointments and lotions to aid skin conditions and kill bacteria. It provides a cooling sensation to the skin, making it ideal for mixing with bath water to escape oppressive summer heat. It works well to repel and kill unwanted insects.

PRECAUTIONS

Camphor oil is toxic when ingested. Even small amounts of the oil can be poisonous, and produce symptoms such as extreme thirst, vomiting, and dizziness. The oil should be diluted before applying topically.

CANNABIS

BOTANICAL NAME: *CANNABIS SATIVA*

No doubt the first thing that comes to mind when we think of cannabis is the recreational drug marijuana; but the oil derived from the flowering cannabis plant is prized for its medicinal benefits. The plant has been found in the graves of ancient Europeans, and is mentioned in various texts written by ancient Egyptians, Indians, and Greeks. Cannabis was used in Chinese medicine as far back as AD 100, and the second-century Chinese surgeon Hua Tuo is the first person known to use the plant as an anesthetic. Although the benefits of the plant have been known for millennia, its association with drug use can make the non-psychoactive essential oil hard to find.

THERAPEUTIC PROPERTIES

Reduces stress and anxiety; pain reliever; improves quality of sleep.

USED FOR

There are hundreds of chemical compounds in cannabis that work together to give the oil many calming, stress-relieving properties. This makes it ideal for people who suffer with anxiety or insomnia. It may also give relief for inflammatory conditions.

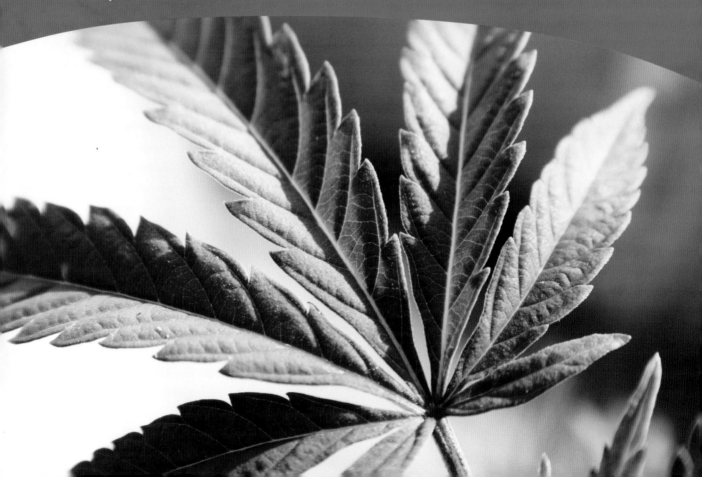

CARAWAY

BOTANICAL NAME: *CARUM CARVI*

Caraway, a biennial plant native to Asia, Europe, and North Africa, is no doubt best known for its culinary use. With its licorice-like flavor and aroma, the spice is commonly used in breads, desserts, and liquors throughout many world cultures. Fossilized caraway seeds have been found at Neolithic and Mesolithic archeological sites, proving that the spice has been in use for at least 8,000 years! Its use in folk medicine—especially as a digestive aid—has been documented since the time of ancient Egypt and Rome. Caraway's strong aroma comes from its essential oil, which is distilled from the seeds and used to fragrance soaps, lotions, and perfumes.

THERAPEUTIC PROPERTIES

Mildly antiseptic; antihistamine; excellent for easing digestion; insect repellent; used as a fragrance.

USED FOR

Caraway can help prevent both internal and external infections, and can be used as a natural antihistamine. Its usefulness as a digestive aid has been known for millennia, as it helps to ease indigestion and heartburn, speeds up digestion, and protects the stomach from ulcers. Historically, caraway has been used as a moth repellent. The oil is frequently used to fragrance soaps, perfumes, and lotions.

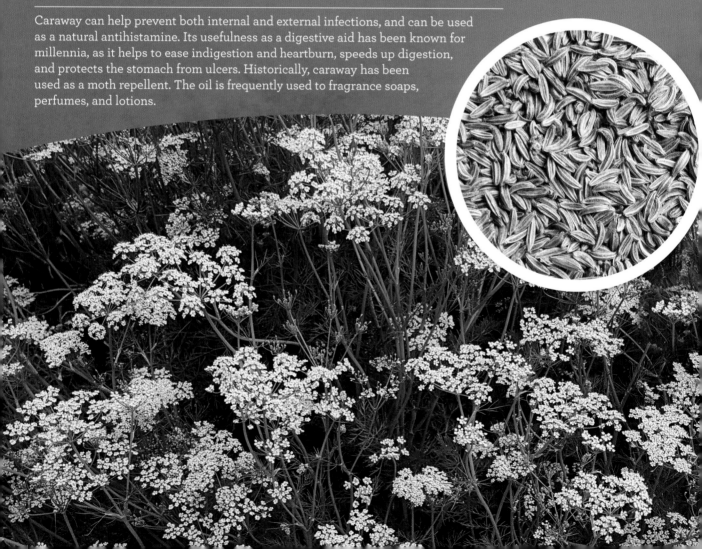

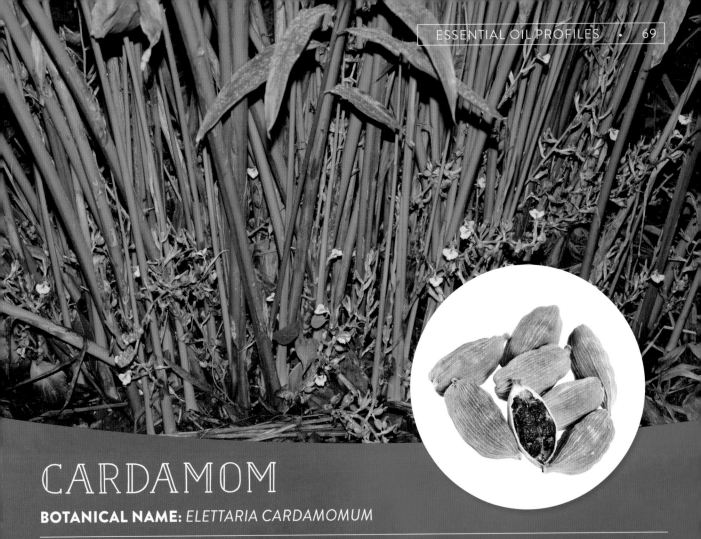

CARDAMOM

BOTANICAL NAME: *ELETTARIA CARDAMOMUM*

If you've ever sipped a cup of spicy chai tea or enjoyed Arabic coffee, they were probably flavored with a healthy dose of cardamom. The third most expensive spice in the world—only vanilla and saffron surpass it—cardamom is native to India; but it is surprisingly widespread in Nordic countries, as well, where it is used in traditional sweet buns and cakes. The spice may have found its way to Scandinavia when Vikings encountered it in Constantinople. And today, Swedes use 60 percent more cardamom than Americans. But the rest of the world should take a cue from Scandinavia: because the deliciously fragrant spice is just as at home in the world of essential oils as it is in the culinary world!

THERAPEUTIC PROPERTIES

Promotes digestion and relieves stomach upset; excellent for aromatherapy; can be used in place of the ground seeds in recipes.

USED FOR

Cardamom has soothing properties that make it great for aiding digestion and calming stomach upset. Try inhaling the scent on car or boat trips to ward off motion sickness. Used in aromatherapy, cardamom helps to relieve anxiety and promote feelings of calm. If a recipe calls for cardamom, the essential oil can be used in place of ground cardamom—a drop or two should be all you need!

CARROT SEED

BOTANICAL NAME: *DAUCUS CAROTA*

Carrot seed essential oil is derived from the seeds of the wild, rather than the domestic, carrot. This flowering plant is related to the common domesticated carrot found in grocery stores. It is also known as Queen Anne's Lace. Carrots trace their roots back to central Asia, where they were originally grown exclusively for their leaves and seeds. In fact, many of the vegetable's relatives—including parsley, cilantro, dill, and cumin—are still grown for the same reason today. Carrot seed was prized in ancient times for its ability to aid digestion and soothe stomach ailments, and today is considered one of the most underrated essential oils on the market.

THERAPEUTIC PROPERTIES

Antioxidant, antiseptic, antiviral; can aid digestion; useful in aromatherapy; anti-parasitic.

USED FOR

Carrot seed oil can be applied topically, either on its own or mixed with lotion or face cream, to rejuvenate skin or help ward off infections. When ingested, it may help fight infections of the mouth or digestive system, and can help treat colds, the flu, and bronchitis. Its soothing aroma helps relieve stress and anxiety when used in aromatherapy. The oil even helps kill intestinal parasites, but is safely consumed by humans.

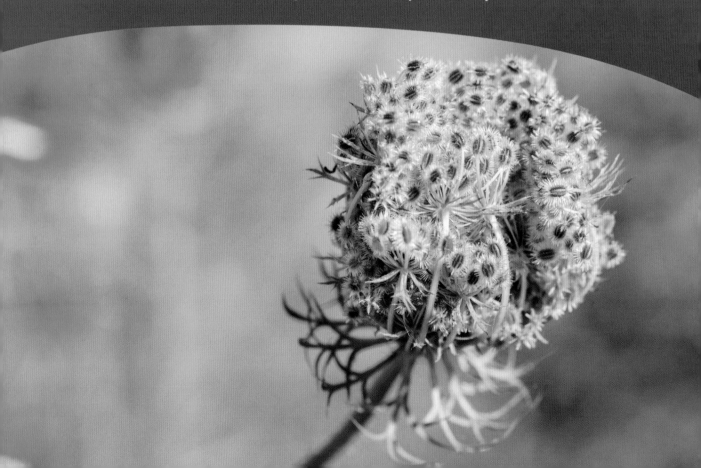

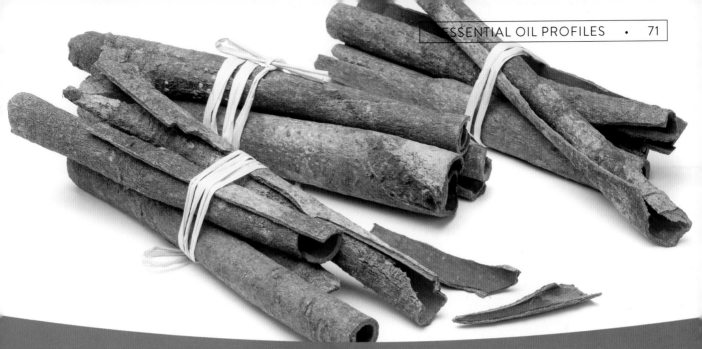

CASSIA

BOTANICAL NAME: *CINNAMONUM CASSIA*

Native to China, cassia is sometimes called "Chinese cinnamon," and is very similar to Ceylon cinnamon—also known as "true" cinnamon. But cassia is actually the most common kind of cinnamon sold in the United States. The dried bark of this evergreen tree has the familiar spicy scent so ubiquitous in a multitude of food and drinks throughout the world. But beyond its obvious worth as a flavoring agent, cassia essential oil has been employed medicinally as far back as biblical times. And in traditional Chinese medicine, the spice is considered one of the 50 fundamental herbs in the practice.

THERAPEUTIC PROPERTIES

Antibacterial; analgesic; helps treat diarrhea; insect repellent; may help lower blood sugar; can be used in cooking.

USED FOR

Cassia has antibacterial properties that can prevent infections in minor cuts or scrapes. It is a warming oil, which makes it excellent for improving circulation and relieving pain caused by arthritis or sore muscles. The oil has been used for centuries as a cure for diarrhea and to promote healthy digestion. Cassia can be used to repel insects—especially as a mosquito repellent. Many studies have suggested that cassia can help lower blood sugar, making it a good oil to have on hand for diabetics. Just like cardamom, cassia oil can be used in place of the ground spice in your favorite recipes.

PRECAUTIONS

Because of its warming properties, cassia can irritate the skin or cause allergic reactions. It's best to do a patch test before using. Ingesting too much of the oil can be harmful to the liver, so always use in minute amounts. Since it may lower blood sugar, diabetics who are on medication should be sure to closely monitor blood sugar to be sure it doesn't dip too low.

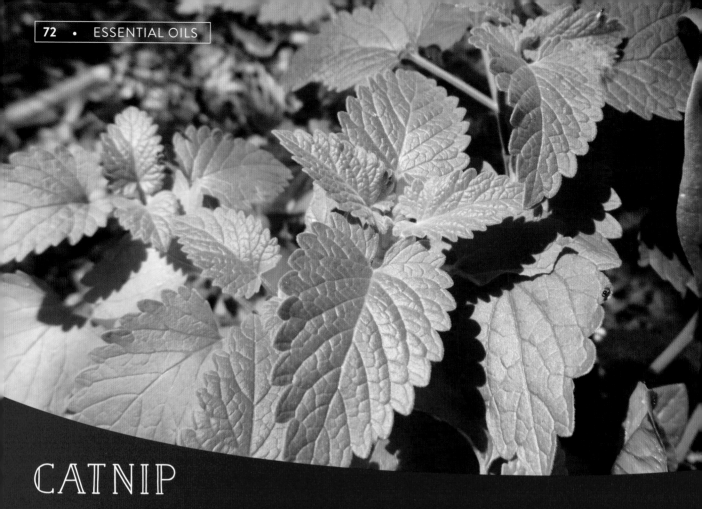

CATNIP

BOTANICAL NAME: *NEPETA CATARIA*

Native to Europe, Africa, and Asia, catnip is best known for being irresistible to our feline friends. But the herbaceous plant has many beneficial qualities that should make it irresistible to people, as well! Unlike the energizing effect it has on cats, catnip has a calming, sedative effect on humans. Ancient Romans took note of this benefit and used the plant in cooking, medicine, and catnip-infused tea. French sailors also enjoyed catnip tea before Chinese tea was readily available. Eventually, the herb was used throughout Europe to promote calm and to aid digestion. And by the 18th century, the herb made its way across the Atlantic, where Native Americans began using it for medicinal purposes.

THERAPEUTIC PROPERTIES

Anti-spasmodic, astringent, sedative; useful as an insect repellent.

USED FOR

Catnip is popular in many calming teas, and drinking it before bedtime can help promote a more restful night's sleep. The essential oil can help to relieve muscle and intestinal cramps, and helps to tone and tighten skin when applied topically. Catnip has even been shown to be more effective at repelling insects than the harmful chemical repellent DEET.

CEDARWOOD

BOTANICAL NAME: *CEDRUS DEODARA OR C. ATLANTICA*

The ancient Egyptians used cedar as a preservative and for embalming, in cosmetics, and as incense. Cedar is included in men's colognes and aftershaves and is used to make cigar boxes, cedar chests, and panel closets. Cedar wood and its essential oil make clothes smell great, and on a practical level, they repel wool moths. You won't find true cedar of Lebanon oil because of the shortage of trees, but Tibetan or Himalayan cedarwood (*C. deodara,* meaning "god tree"), and Atlas cedarwood (*C. atlantica*) have similar scents. The modern source of most "cedarwood" oil is juniper (*Juniperus virginiana*), known as "red cedar." Don't confuse cedarwood with thuja or cedar leaf (*Thuja occidentalis*).

THERAPEUTIC PROPERTIES

Antiseptic, astringent; brings on menstruation, clears mucus, sedates nerves, stimulates circulation.

USED FOR

Inhale the steam of cedarwood essential oil to treat respiratory infections and clear congestion. Add a few drops to a sitz bath to ease the pain and irritation of urinary infections and to cure the infection more quickly. Applied to oily skin, cedarwood essential oil is an astringent that dries and helps clear acne. Incorporate it into a facial wash, spritzer, or other cosmetic (10 drops of essential oil per ounce of preparation). Added to a salve (15 drops of essential oil per ounce of salve), it relieves dermatitis and, in some cases, eczema and psoriasis. Add two drops of essential oil to every ounce of shampoo or hair conditioner to ease dandruff.

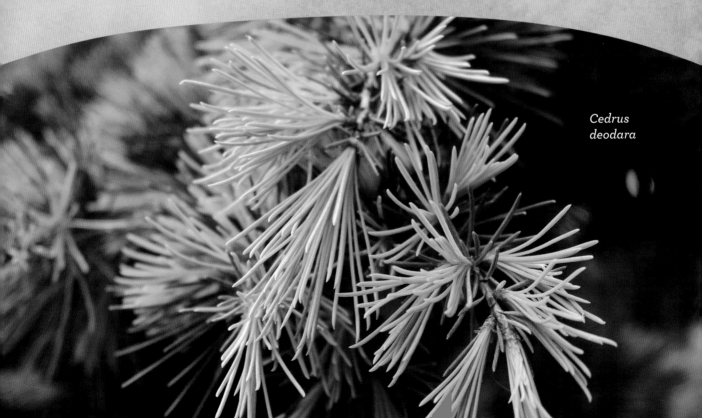

Cedrus deodara

CELERY SEED

BOTANICAL NAME: *APIUM GRAVEOLENS*

Many a delicious dish begins with a few stalks of celery: the French can't make their *mirepoix* without it, and the "holy trinity" of Cajun cuisine includes celery, onions, and bell peppers. But celery has never been content to merely flavor the culinary world. The leafy vegetable has also been prized for its medicinal benefits since antiquity. In Chinese and Ayurvedic medicine, celery was used to treat everything from colds and flu to high blood pressure and kidney stones. Even Hippocrates—the "Father of Medicine"—was known to prescribe celery to his patients. Although all parts of the vegetable itself contain essential oil, it is the seeds that produce the most potent variety.

THERAPEUTIC PROPERTIES

Anti-inflammatory; helps to lower blood pressure; eases digestion and prevents ulcers; insect repellent.

USED FOR

Celery seed oil works well as an anti-inflammatory massage oil to relieve achy muscles or pain from arthritis. It has a relaxing effect on the nervous system, which can help lower blood pressure. Celery seed helps to prevent indigestion and diarrhea, and may protect the stomach against ulcers. It works well as a natural insecticide, and is especially useful for warding off mosquitoes.

PRECAUTIONS

Since celery seed oil may lower blood pressure, those with already low blood pressure should avoid it. It should not be used by pregnant women.

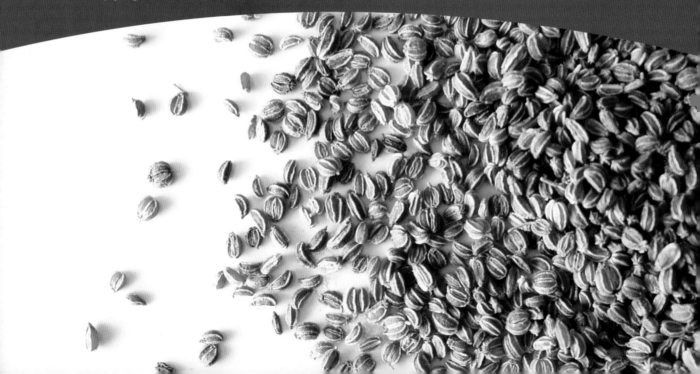

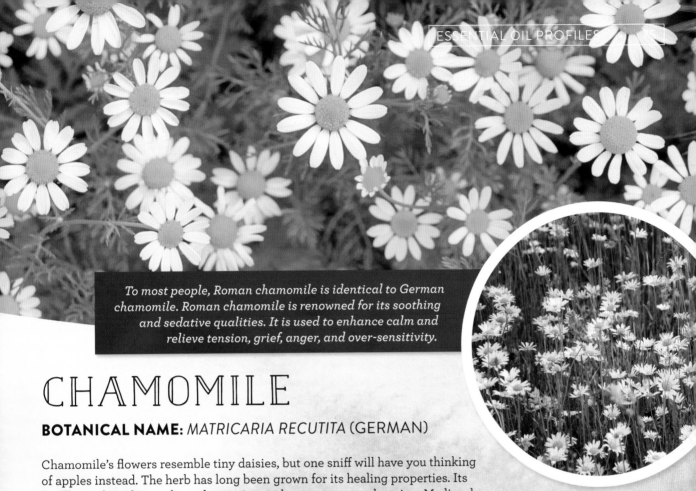

To most people, Roman chamomile is identical to German chamomile. Roman chamomile is renowned for its soothing and sedative qualities. It is used to enhance calm and relieve tension, grief, anger, and over-sensitivity.

CHAMOMILE

BOTANICAL NAME: *MATRICARIA RECUTITA* (GERMAN)

Chamomile's flowers resemble tiny daisies, but one sniff will have you thinking of apples instead. The herb has long been grown for its healing properties. Its smell was thought to relieve depression and to encourage relaxation. Medieval monks planted raised garden beds of chamomile, and those who were sad or depressed lay on them as therapy. Chamomile also was once a "strewing herb," spread on bare floors so that the scent was released when people walked on it. Drinking chamomile tea made from the flowers stimulates appetite before meals; after meals it settles the stomach. Roman chamomile (*Camaemelum nobile*, formerly *Anthemis nobilis*) yields a pale yellow essential oil that is an anti-inflammatory. When German chamomile (left) is distilled, a chemical reaction produces the deep blue-green chamazulene that is even more potent an anti-inflammatory.

Inhaling chamomile tea's aroma relaxes both the mind and the body. Research studies show that chamomile relaxes emotions, muscles, and even brain waves. It eases the emotional ups and downs of PMS, menopause, and hyperactivity in children. It also helps control the pain of bruises, stiff joints, headaches, sore muscles, menstrual and digestive system cramping, as well as the pain and swelling of sprains and some allergic reactions. Chamomile is mild enough to ease a baby's colic and calm it for sleep. It is especially soothing in a massage oil, as a compress, or in a bath. Make a chamomile room spray by diluting 12 drops of the essential oil per ounce of distilled water. Chamomile is suitable for most complexion types or skin problems, from burns and eczema to varicose veins. It is especially useful for sensitive, puffy, or inflamed conditions. Add it to shampoos to lighten and brighten hair.

THERAPEUTIC PROPERTIES

Anti-inflammatory, antiseptic; promotes digestion, relieves gas and nausea, encourages menstruation, soothes nervous tension, promotes sleep.

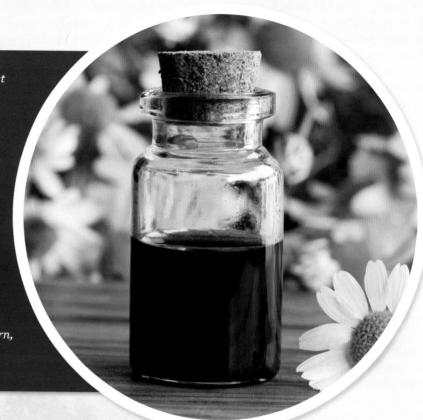

German chamomile is arguably the most healing of the chamomile essential oils. Its striking blue to blue-green color comes from chamazulene. This powerful compound can also be found in a few other essential oils, like blue tansy, wormwood, and yarrow. Chamazulene's healing properties are truly amazing. Thanks to its ability to fight inflammation and infection and promote tissue regeneration, this compound is applicable to just about any common skin condition. Chamazulene is helpful in dealing with eczema, psoriasis, dermatitis, poison ivy, cuts, infections, boils, blisters, warts, insect bites, sunburn, and even deeper tissue ailments, from surface bruises to rheumatic pain.

SACRED CHAMOMILE

Chamomile has been used medicinally for thousands of years. Ancient Egyptians used it to treat nervous afflictions and sleeping problems. Ancient Romans used it to treat skin and respiratory conditions. It takes its name from the Greek word *chamaimelon*, meaning "ground apple." Greek physicians treated intestinal disorders with chamomile. During the Middle Ages it was used to treat a variety of ailments and was also used as a strewing herb—bundles of the plant were simply thrown on the floor where they would be walked over, releasing their scent, repelling vermin, and helping to clear the air. One Anglo-Saxon manuscript tells us that chamomile was one of the "Nine Sacred Herbs." Modern herbalists continue to recommend chamomile for many of its traditional uses.

MOROCCAN CHAMOMILE

Moroccan chamomile essential oil is not from a true chamomile plant, and its chemical constituents are very different from the German and Roman varieties. It is a chamomile-like cousin perennial whose medicinal attributes are not yet fully explored. It is also a relative newcomer to aromatherapy. Due to its intriguingly sweet and fruity aroma, it is used in perfumery and cosmetics. It may have skin-healing and sedative properties. According to some aromatherapists, it may ease sore muscles and joints when used in a massage blend.

CILANTRO

BOTANICAL NAME: *CORIANDRUM SATIVUM*

Cilantro is sometimes called Chinese parsley or coriander. It has an unmistakable scent and flavor that people seem to either love or hate. The ancient Greek word for the herb was *koris*—which was also their name for bed bugs! Cilantro can be found in cuisines around the world, from Mexico to China to India. Remains of the herb have been found at archeological sites in Israel dating back 8,000 years, and it is said to have grown in the famous Hanging Gardens of Babylon. If you've only ever thought of cilantro as a guacamole ingredient, check out some of the essential oil's healthy benefits. Diffused, the essential oil has a bracing, fresh herbal scent that is fantastic for clearing unwanted odors.

THERAPEUTIC PROPERTIES

Antibacterial and antifungal; analgesic; promotes healthy digestion.

USED FOR

Cilantro's antibacterial and antifungal properties make it a great choice to use as a natural deodorant and mouthwash. Simply mix with water, and apply to underarms or swish it around in your mouth to prevent microbial growth. Cilantro can help ease pain caused by toothaches, headaches, or arthritis. The oil helps to aid digestion, especially after overindulging in a meal. Via diffuser, cilantro has an exceptional ability to mitigate the smell of airborne cigarette smoke.

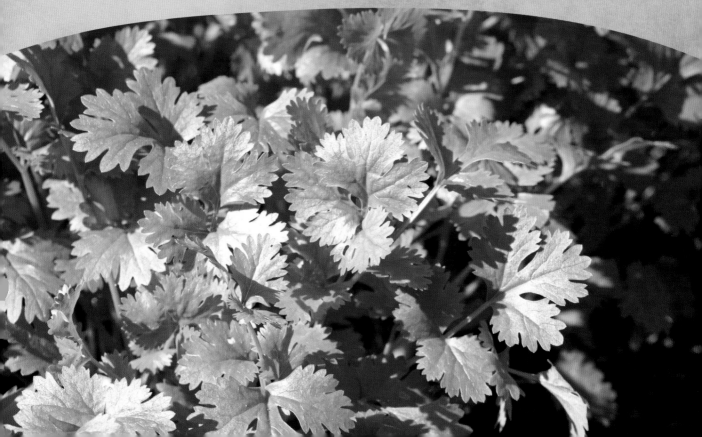

CINNAMON

BOTANICAL NAME: *CINNAMOMUM ZEYLANICUM*

The *zeylanicum* "true" cinnamon starts off as the dry inner bark of a large 20-to-30-foot tree most likely growing in Sri Lanka. The Arabs, Portuguese, Dutch, and British successively controlled trade of this valuable spice. Then, as now, cinnamon flavored mouthwashes, foods, and drinks, and was used as an aphrodisiac. Cinnamon's scent also stirs the appetite, invigorates and "warms" the senses, and may even produce a feeling of joy. There are two main kinds of essential oil made from *zeylanicum*. The oil made from the bark is the most pungently cinnamon-like, while a milder oil is made from the leaves.

THERAPEUTIC PROPERTIES

Antiseptic, digestive, antiviral; relieves muscle spasms and rheumatic pain when used topically.

USED FOR

In general, cinnamon is used as a physical and emotional stimulant. Researchers have found that it reduces drowsiness, irritability, and the pain and number of headaches. In one study, the aroma of cinnamon in the room helped participants to concentrate and perform better. The essential oil and its fragrance help relax tight muscles, ease painful joints, and relieve menstrual cramps.

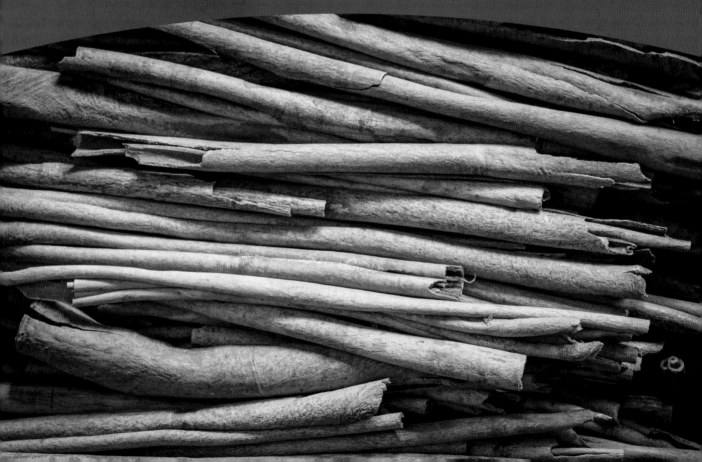

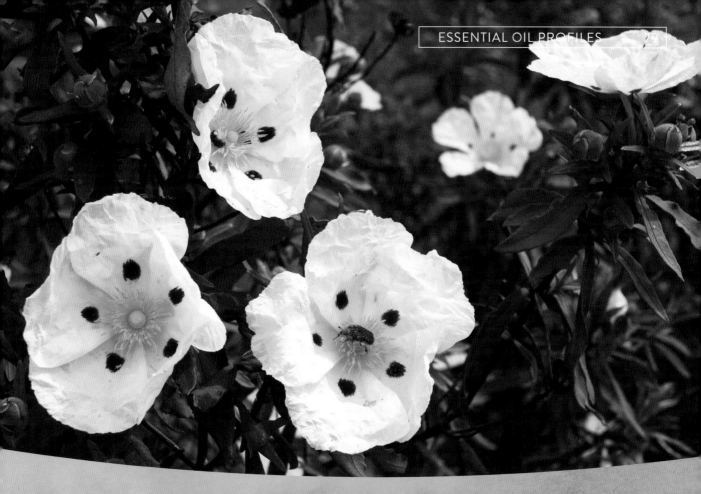

CISTUS

BOTANICAL NAME: *CISTUS LADANIFER*

Cistus, also commonly known as rockrose or labdanum, is a flowering plant found in the Mediterranean region. It has been prized for its amber-like scent since the time of the ancient Egyptians, and is even mentioned in the biblical book of Genesis. In ancient times, shepherds would collect the sweet-smelling resin of the cistus shrub by brushing it off the hair of their goats and sheep, which grazed on the plants. The resin was then used to treat colds, coughs, and arthritis, as well as for incense. By the Middle Ages, the use of the plant had spread to Europe, where it was used to treat wounds and skin ulcers.

THERAPEUTIC PROPERTIES

Antimicrobial, astringent; helps to slow bleeding; useful in aromatherapy.

USED FOR

Cistus is often used to give perfumes a warm, amber note, and is said to promote feelings of calm and peace when used in aromatherapy. It is popular in many skincare products, providing benefits for those struggling with acne, oily skin, eczema, or psoriasis. Cistus can also help to stop bleeding from fresh cuts and scrapes.

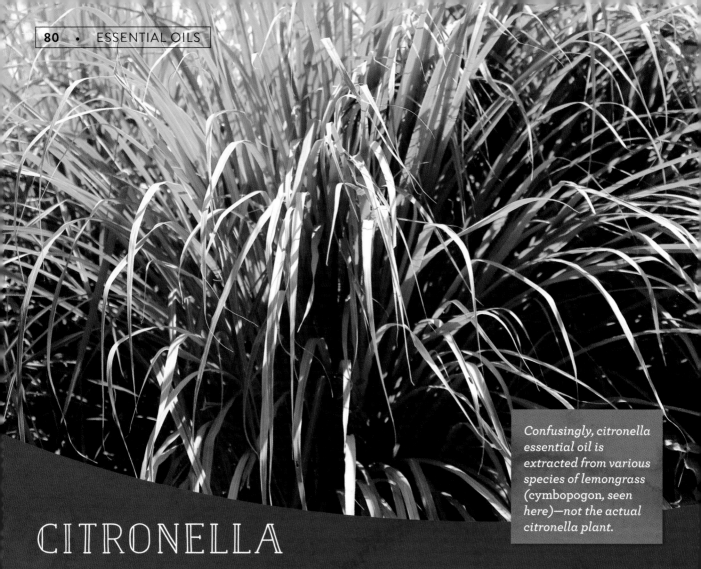

Confusingly, citronella essential oil is extracted from various species of lemongrass (cymbopogon, seen here)—not the actual citronella plant.

CITRONELLA

BOTANICAL NAME: *CYMBOPOGON NARDUS, C. WINTERIANUS*, AND OTHERS

Citronella grass is a type of lemongrass native to tropical Asia. The grass grows to about six and a half feet in length. It is a popular choice for home gardens due to its supposed ability to ward off insects—though some studies have found it ineffective for this use. The oil extracted from the plant's stems and leaves has many other uses as well. In fact, citronella oil has been used in China, Indonesia, and Sri Lanka for centuries for medicinal purposes. Many clinical studies have shown the oil to be an effective antiseptic, making it a natural bug bite remedy.

THERAPEUTIC PROPERTIES

Antiseptic, antimicrobial, antifungal; insect repellent.

USED FOR

The oil continues to be popular as a natural insect repellent, albeit with mixed results. A few drops can be added to coconut oil and then rubbed on like body lotion. It can be used as a skin remedy to help heal bug bites, eczema, or fungal infections. Its fresh scent and antiseptic properties make it an excellent kitchen and bathroom cleaner.

CLARY SAGE

BOTANICAL NAME: *SALVIA SCLAREA*

In ancient times, clary sage was praised as a panacea with the ability to render man immortal. The tea was once thought not only to clear eyesight and the brain, but also to clarify one's intuition and allow one to see more clearly into the future. Simply sniffing the oil before going to bed can produce dramatic dreams and, when you awake, a euphoric state of mind. It was an important ingredient in one of the most popular European cordials. Along with elderflowers, it still flavors high quality Muscatel wine and Italian vermouth. Distilled from the flowering tops and leaves of a three-foot-tall perennial, clary sage now is produced mostly for flavoring a large variety of foods.

THERAPEUTIC PROPERTIES

Antidepressant, anti-inflammatory, astringent, deodorant; decreases gas and indigestion, brings on menstruation, relaxes muscles and nerves, and lowers blood pressure.

USED FOR

Added to a massage oil or used in a compress, clary sage eases muscle and nervous tension and pain. Its relaxing action can reduce muscle spasms and asthma attacks and lower blood pressure. Especially good for female ailments, it helps one cope better with menstrual cramps or PMS and has established itself as a premier remedy for menopausal hot flashes. Improve your complexion by adding it to creams, especially if you have acne or thin, wrinkled, or inflamed skin.

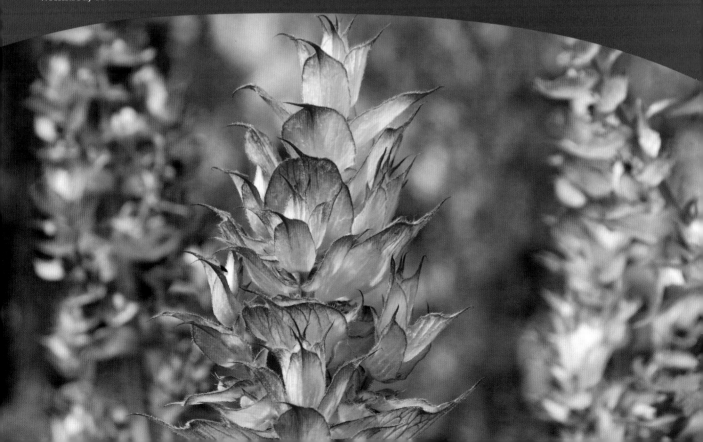

CLOVE

BOTANICAL NAME: *SYZYGIUM AROMATICUM*

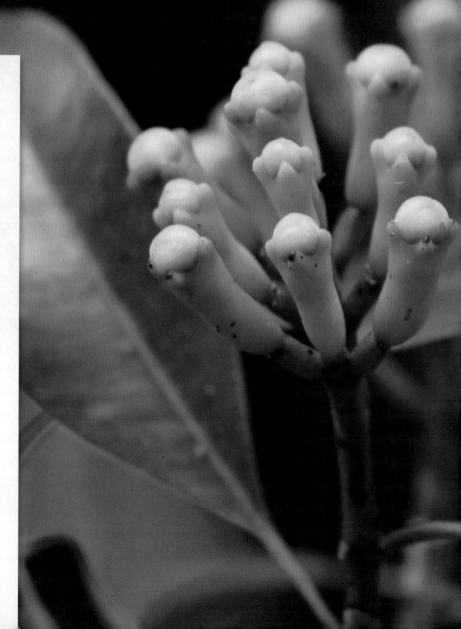

The flower buds are picked and then sorted. The buds are dried on mats in the sun for about three days.

In ancient China, courtiers at the Han court held cloves in their mouths to freshen their breath before they had an audience with the emperor. Today, cloves are still used to sweeten breath. Modern dental preparations numb tooth and gum pain and quell infection with clove essential oil or its main constituent, eugenol. Simply inhaling the fragrance was once said to improve eyesight and fend off the plague. Clove's scent developed a reputation, now backed by science, for being stimulating. The fragrance was also believed to be an aphrodisiac. Cloves were so valuable that a Frenchman risked his life to steal a clove tree from the Dutch colonies in Indonesia and plant it in French ground. Once established, the slender evergreen trees bear buds for at least a century. The familiar clove buds used to poke hams and flavor mulled wine are picked while still unripe and dried before being shipped or distilled into essential oil.

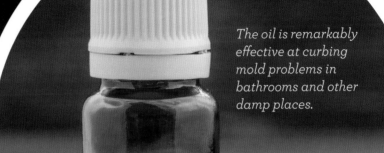

The oil is remarkably effective at curbing mold problems in bathrooms and other damp places.

As an antiseptic and pain reliever, clove essential oil relieves toothaches, flu, colds, and bronchial congestion. But don't try to use it straight on an infant's gums for teething as is often suggested, or you may end up with a screaming baby because it tastes so strong and hot. Instead mix only two drops of clove oil in at least a teaspoon of vegetable oil. It can still be hot, however, so try it in your own mouth first. Then apply it directly to the baby's gums. In a heating liniment, clove essential oil helps sore muscles and arthritis. Mix 30 drops of clove essential oil in one ounce of apple cider vinegar, shake well, and dab on athlete's foot. Researchers have found that the spicy aroma of clove reduces drowsiness, irritability, and headaches.

PRECAUTIONS

The essential oil irritates skin and mucous membranes, so be sure to dilute it before use. Clove leaf is almost pure eugenol; do not use it in aromatherapy preparations.

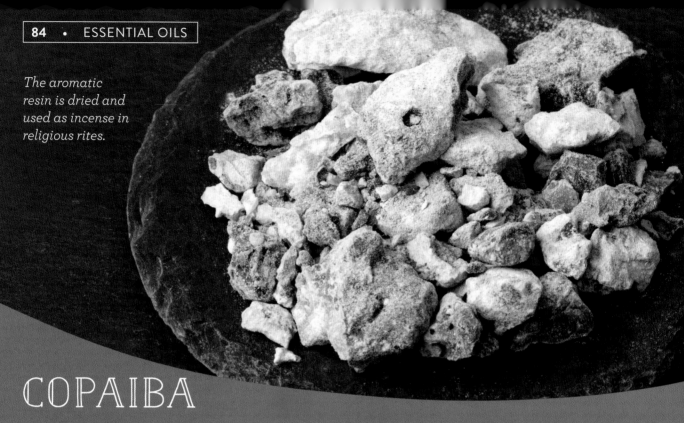

The aromatic resin is dried and used as incense in religious rites.

COPAIBA

BOTANICAL NAME: *COPAIFERA LANGSDORFFII, C. RETICULATA,* AND OTHERS

Grown in South American tropical rain forests, the tree that yields copaiba oil is often called the "diesel tree" because the oil can be used for fuel. Many people have found the oil useful for making lacquer and varnish, and it is also popularly used by artists for oil painting and pottery. But indigenous people in Brazil have used the oil medicinally since at least the 16th century, and 21st century studies have lent credence to their practices: the oil has been found to have anti-inflammatory, antiseptic, and anti-hemorrhagic properties. The popularity of this oil has been spreading around the world, and the production of copaiba oil now makes up 95 percent of Brazil's oil-resin production industry.

THERAPEUTIC PROPERTIES

Anti-inflammatory, antibacterial, astringent; may help to reduce blood pressure.

USED FOR

Copaiba oil is popularly used to tone and tighten skin, and reduce the appearance of scars and stretch marks. Its anti-inflammatory properties also make it a great choice for calming acne. It helps to to reduce pain caused by arthritis, headaches, muscle cramps, and injuries, either used as aromatherapy or applied topically. Some have described the scent of copaiba oil as being sweet like honey, and breathing in the soothing scent may help to lower blood pressure.

PRECAUTIONS

While copaiba oil is safe to ingest in minute amounts, consuming too much can cause stomach pain and symptoms similar to food poisoning. Use very sparingly.

CORIANDER

BOTANICAL NAME: *CORIANDRUM SATIVUM*

The coriander plant is synonymous with cilantro (see page 77). This native to west Asia, Europe, and the eastern Mediterranean has been used for centuries as an aphrodisiac, to lift spirits, assist digestion, and restore calm. The seeds were reputedly found in the tomb of the Egyptian pharaoh Rameses II. It is now cultivated across the globe.

The essential oil of coriander is not distilled from the herb, but rather from the seeds. It has a pungent and refreshing aroma, with sweet and slightly woody and peppery overtones. Aromatherapists note that it has the ability to quell bad moods, calm frayed nerves, and promote feelings of relaxation.

THERAPEUTIC PROPERTIES

Analgesic, antispasmodic, carminative, deodorant; relieves anxiety and depression.

USED FOR

Diffused, coriander can be a powerful and uplifting mood enhancer. It relieves anxiety, insomnia, lethargy, and weariness. A few diluted drops, taken internally after a large meal, promote digestion.

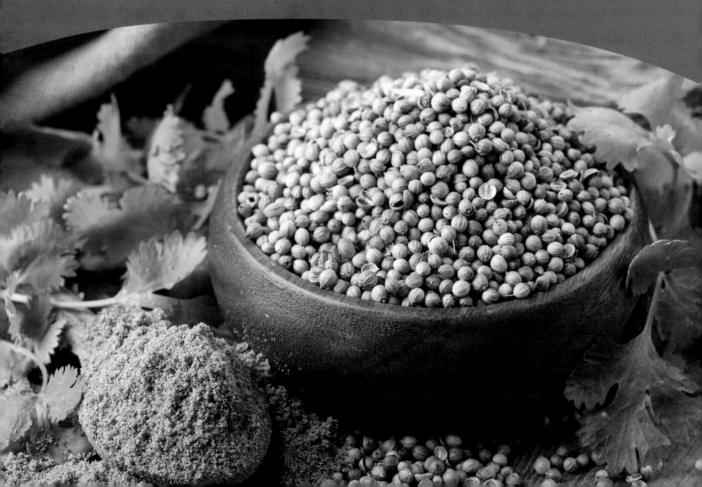

CYPRESS

BOTANICAL NAME: *CUPRESSUS SEMPERVIRENS*

Greeks say that cypress clears the mind during stressful times and comforts mourners. Cypress stanches bleeding (Hippocrates recommended it for hemorrhoids) and the Chinese chewed its small cones, rich in essential oils and astringents, to heal bleeding gums. The greenish essential oil is distilled from the tree's needles or twigs and sometimes from its cones.

THERAPEUTIC PROPERTIES

Antiseptic, astringent, deodorant; relieves rheumatic pain, relaxes muscle spasms and cramping, stops bleeding, constricts blood vessels.

USED FOR

Cypress's specialty is treating circulation problems, such as low blood pressure, poor circulation, varicose veins, and hemorrhoids. Because it helps heal broken capillaries and also discourages fluid retention, it is a favored essential oil at menopause. For these uses, add 8 drops to every ounce of cream or lotion and apply gently to the afflicted region a couple of times a day. You can also alleviate laryngitis, spasmodic coughing, and lung congestion just by putting a drop on your pillow. Because of its astringent, antiseptic, and deodorant properties, dilute about 6 drops of cypress essential oil in vinegar or aloe vera for an oily complexion or to reduce excessive sweating.

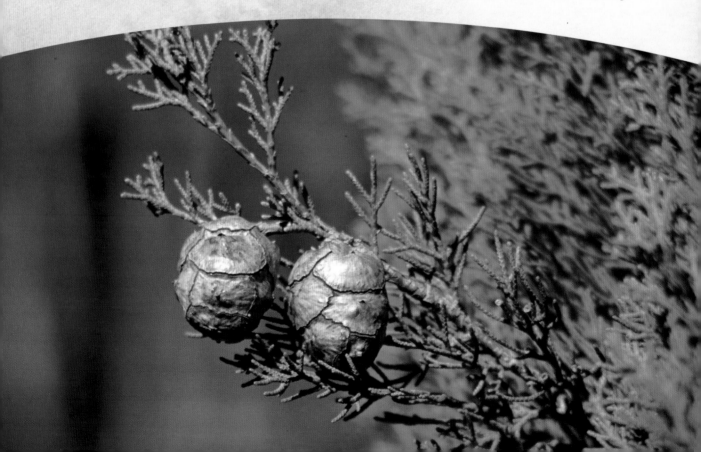

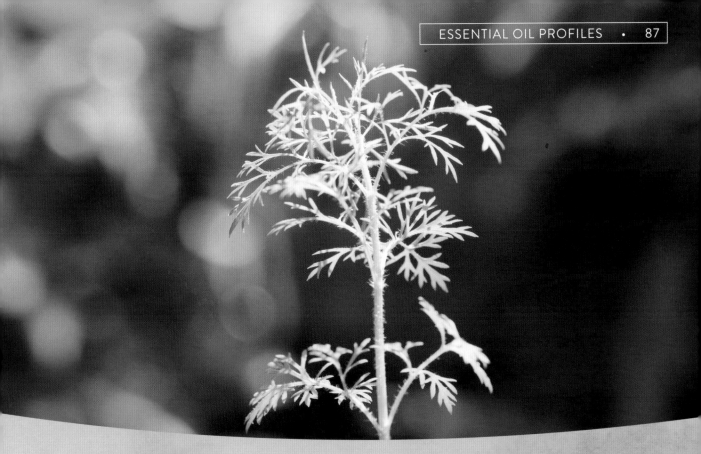

DAVANA

BOTANICAL NAME: *ARTEMISIA PALLENS*

Traditionally, the davana plant has been used in religious ceremonies in its native India, where it is offered to the god Shiva by Hindu devotees. But this flowering member of the daisy family has also been used in Indian folk medicine for hundreds of years to treat diabetes and high blood pressure. In fact, davana is offered to Shiva exactly for this reason: to show gratitude for the medicinal properties the plant possesses. In modern times, davana oil is especially prized for use in perfumes, because of its unique tendency to smell differently depending on the person wearing it. This results in a truly one-of-a-kind fragrance for perfume aficionados!

THERAPEUTIC PROPERTIES

Antimicrobial; helps to relieve coughs and congestion; may help to alleviate depression and anxiety; perfume additive.

USED FOR

Davana oil has been shown to rupture the protective cover of viruses, making it an effective remedy against colds and flu. It also fights bacterial infections in the body or on the skin, and can be used to disinfect surfaces in kitchens, bathrooms, and other rooms of your home. When used in aromatherapy, the soothing fragrance helps to lower blood pressure and may even help to relax the nervous system. The oil is used in the manufacture of perfumes, cosmetics, and some foods and beverages.

DILL

BOTANICAL NAME: *ANETHUM GRAVEOLENS*

Dill's obvious claim to fame is its inclusion in pickle recipes. What deli sandwich would be complete without a dill pickle on the side? The biennial herb was called *Anethon* by the ancient Egyptians, Greeks, and Romans—its botanical name was derived from this word. Our word comes from the Old English *dylle*, which means "to lull." A fitting description, as dill essential oil is known to have soothing, calming properties. In fact, Romans used to rub themselves with dill oil before heading into battle, to calm their nerves! You may not be charging into battle any time soon, but dill's many benefits may convince you to add it to your essential oil arsenal.

THERAPEUTIC PROPERTIES

Antibacterial; relieves muscle spasms; aids digestion; sedative.

USED FOR

Dill oil can help prevent infections, both internal and external, and can even prevent lice infestations if applied to the scalp. The oil can relieve muscle spasms and calm cramps. It has been used for millennia as a way to support healthy digestion, and helps alleviate constipation, gas, and indigestion. When used in aromatherapy, its calming, sedative properties help relieve anxiety and promote a good night's sleep.

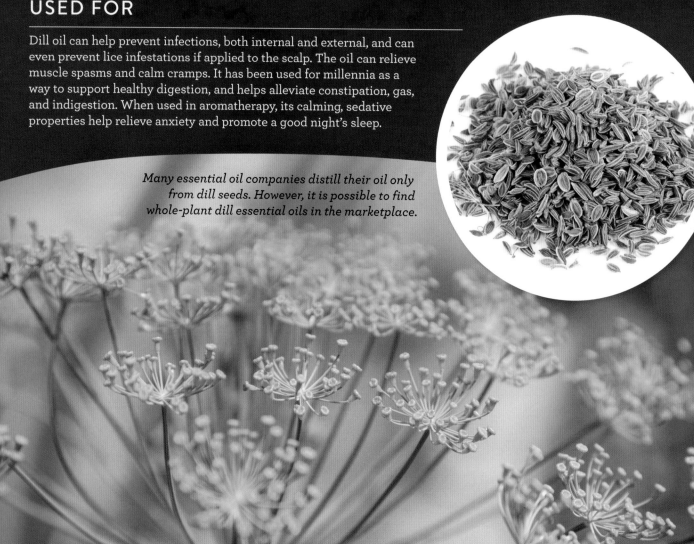

Many essential oil companies distill their oil only from dill seeds. However, it is possible to find whole-plant dill essential oils in the marketplace.

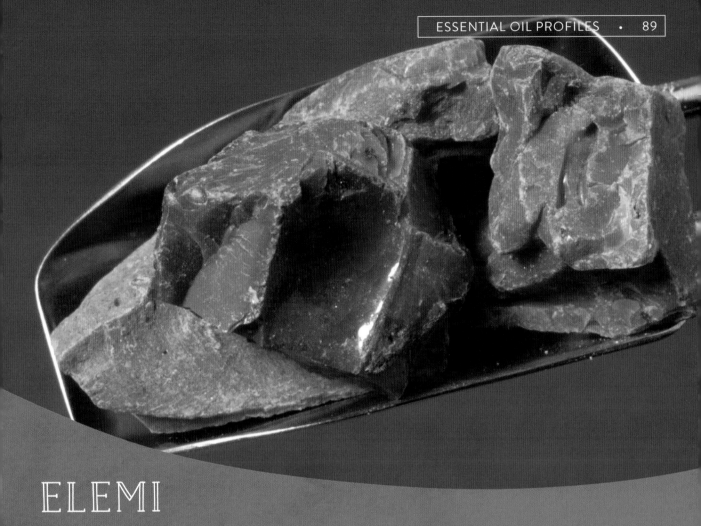

ELEMI

BOTANICAL NAME: *CANARIUM LUZONICUM*

Elemi is derived from a tree found in the tropical forests of the Philippines. It belongs to the same botanical family as frankincense and myrrh. Between January and June, when the leaves of the tree are budding, the gum resin is harvested from the trees. The essential oil is then steam extracted from the resin, producing a product with a peppery, lemony scent. By the 7th century, elemi oil was being used in religious ceremonies in China; but it was the explorer Magellan's discovery of the Philippines in 1521 that helped introduce the oil to Europe and the Middle East. By the 18th century, elemi had found a home among other therapeutic oils used in the West, where it was considered an essential medicinal ingredient.

THERAPEUTIC PROPERTIES

Antiseptic; analgesic; helps alleviate cold and flu symptoms; perfume additive.

USED FOR

Elemi's antiseptic properties help to protect against infections of many kinds, including bacterial, fungal, and viral. It helps to reduce pain caused by injuries, headaches, or arthritis. It helps to ease breathing and reduce congestion due to colds and coughs.

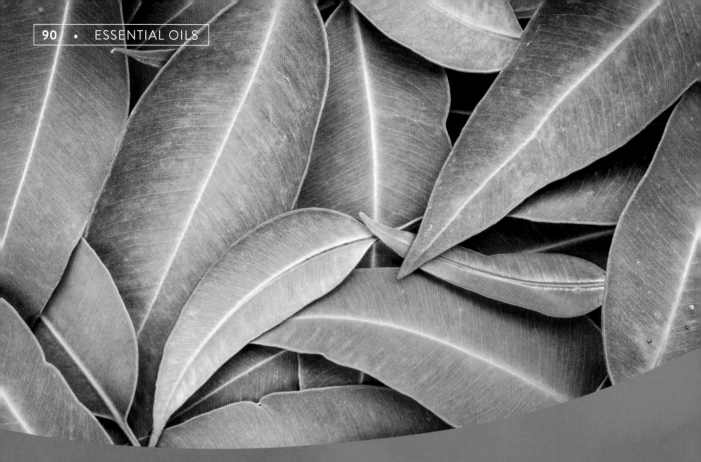

EUCALYPTUS

BOTANICAL NAME: *EUCALYPTUS GLOBULUS*

Eucalyptus or "gum" trees originated in Australia and Tasmania, but they are now found in subtropical regions all over the globe. Eucalyptus' thick, long, bluish-green leaves are distilled to provide essential oil. Blue gum eucalyptus, the most widely cultivated variety, provides most of the commercially available oil, although with more than 600 species, there are a variety of scents. Aromatherapists sometimes favor the more relaxing qualities and pleasant scent of the lemony *E. citriodora*. A very inexpensive oil, eucalyptus is used liberally to scent aftershaves and colognes and as an antiseptic in mouthwashes and household cleansers.

THERAPEUTIC PROPERTIES

Antibacterial, antiviral, deodorant; clears mucous from the lungs; as a liniment it relieves rheumatic, arthritic, and other types of pain.

USED FOR

It is the most popular essential oil steam for relieving sinus and lung congestion such as asthma. Inhale the steam, add one or two drops of oil to a compress, or put three or four drops in your bath. Especially appropriate for skin eruptions and oily complexions, it is also used for acne, herpes, and chicken pox. For a homemade preparation, mix eucalyptus essential oil with an equal amount of apple cider vinegar and dab on problem areas. This mix can also be used as an antiseptic on wounds, boils, and insect bites.

FENNEL

BOTANICAL NAME: *FOENICULUM VULGARE*

Known for its licorice-like flavor, fennel, a member of the carrot family, is native to the Mediterranean. But the flowering plant is now found all over the world, including Europe and the United States, and is coveted for both its taste and its therapeutic benefits. The herb was noted for its medicinal properties as far back as the 10th century, and even the poet Henry Wadsworth Longfellow wrote about fennel's "wondrous powers." Today, the herb is commonly used in foods, drinks, and cosmetics, but it is especially prized for its effectiveness at treating digestive issues.

THERAPEUTIC PROPERTIES

Antimicrobial; relieves digestive upset; may aid in weight loss.

USED FOR

Fennel oil can help to heal minor cuts and scrapes and prevent infection, and fights free radical damage in the body. The oil is especially useful for relieving digestive issues, including abdominal cramps, irritable bowel syndrome, gas, constipation, and diarrhea. Fennel oil may boost metabolism and suppress appetite, making it an excellent addition to a weight loss plan.

PRECAUTIONS

Heavy doses of fennel oil can have narcotic effects, causing hallucinations or convulsions. It is recommended that anyone with a history of seizures avoid using fennel oil.

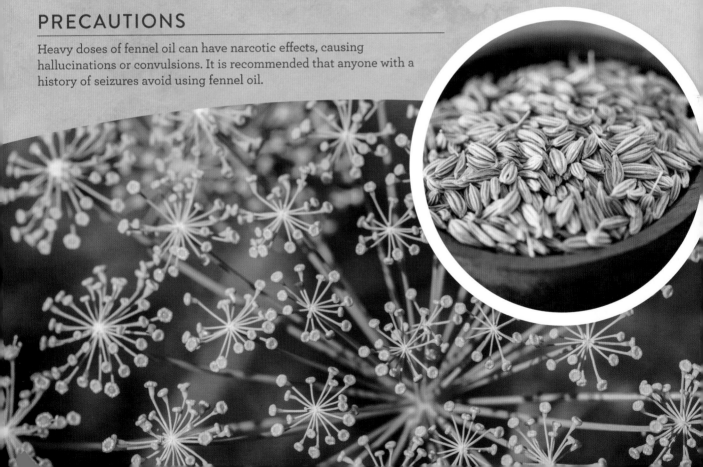

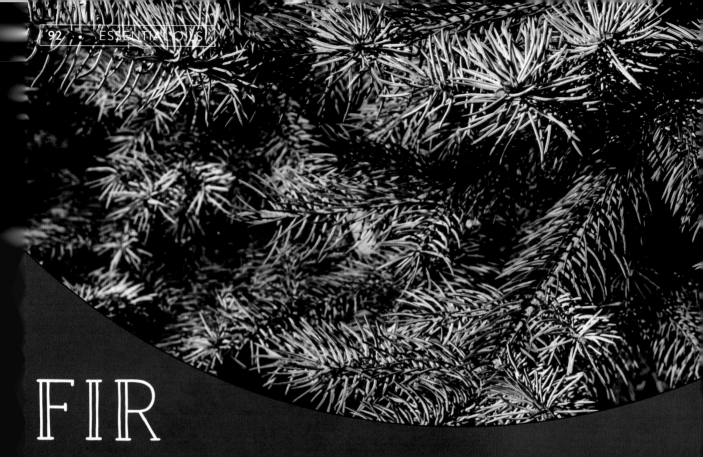

FIR

BOTANICAL NAME: *ABIES ALBA* AND OTHERS

For centuries, fir boughs were scattered over floors of churches and houses during winter, providing a clean, scented covering. Perhaps long ago, people realized that the uplifting fragrance helped overcome winter blues and encouraged feelings of contentment and joy.

Fir essential oil is distilled from the twigs or needles of many different conifers, yielding a rich variety of fragrances. The Canadian Balsam (*A. balsamea*) and Siberian firs (*A. siberica*) have an especially pleasant, forest-like scent, while the white fir (*A. concolor*) is excellent in massage blends. You may find other fir essential oils with similar uses and scent profiles, such as the Fraser (*A. fraseri*), Nordmann (*A. nordmanniana*), and Grand (*A. grandis*).

THERAPEUTIC PROPERTIES

Antibacterial, deodorant; relieves pain and coughing, clears mucous from the lungs, kills mold.

USED FOR

Fir essential oils soothe muscle and rheumatism pain and increase poor circulation when used in a massage oil or when added to a liniment or bath. They also help prevent bronchial and urinary infections and reduce coughing, including that caused by bronchitis and asthma. The best ways to utilize the essential oil are either through inhalation or via a chest rub. It is occasionally added to a salve or other skin preparation as an antiseptic for skin infections. An aromatherapy alarm clock from Japan uses the forest scent of pine or fir along with eucalyptus for

SIBERIAN FIR

Siberian fir is an excellent addition to blends designed to fight colds, flu, and respiratory problems. It is effective in massage blends used for muscle aches, joint inflammation, and arthritis. In aromatherapy, Siberian fir is considered a particularly bracing oil—it is suggested as a supporting fragrance for those undergoing stressful life transitions.

GRAND FIR

The Grand fir is one of the species harvested for the domestic Christmas tree market. It's no surprise then that its essential oil has the classic conifer smell that many associate with the holidays. The essential oil works well in scented candles, deodorizing sprays, and air fresheners. In aromatherapy, Grand fir is known for fighting fatigue, depression, and general listlessness.

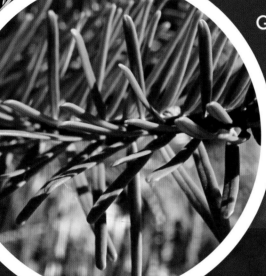

Grand fir

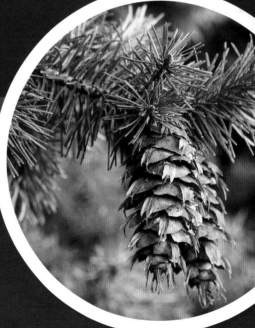

Douglas fir

DOUGLAS FIR

To many people, the Douglas fir is the classic Christmas tree. It has a crisp, uplifting smell that makes it another great candidate for diffusion, steam baths, and other air freshening applications. It also has disinfectant properties that make it useful in cleaners and soaps. As with Grand fir, its use in aromatherapy contributes to a positive, uplifting environment.

BALSAM FIR

Compared to other fir essential oils, balsam fir is notably mild, grassy, and well-rounded in aroma. But it still has that classic outdoorsy forest fragrance that has such a positive impact on mood and emotional equilibrium. Topically, balsam fir has strong anti-inflammatory action. It's another great addition to massage oils created for sore muscles. It is specifically recommended for breaking up persistent chest colds, coughs, and bronchial problems.

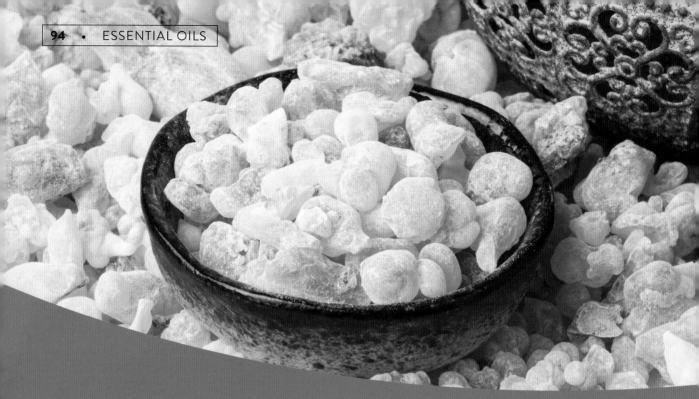

FRANKINCENSE

BOTANICAL NAME: *BOSWELLIA CARTERI*

The frankincense burned as church incense today is the same as that used by ancient peoples who inhabited the Middle East and North Africa. Eventually the use of frankincense spread throughout Europe and eastward into India, and it was burned as an offering to the gods of many cultures.

Aromatherapists and massage practitioners have observed that frankincense's fragrance can deepen breathing, aid relaxation, and cause the lungs to expand. Modern science backs up these observations by showing that, when burned, frankincense releases molecules of trahydrocannabinole, a psychoactive compound that may be responsible for uplifting the spirit. The pale yellow oil is steam distilled from hard "tears" of oleo gum resin.

THERAPEUTIC PROPERTIES

Antiseptic, anti-inflammatory, antifungal, astringent, sedative; clears lung congestion, decreases gas and indigestion, brings on menstruation.

USED FOR

Its antiseptic and skin-healing properties fight bacterial and fungal skin infections and boils. Since it's quite expensive, however, it is usually reserved for the most difficult cases, such as unsightly scars that remain after an infection has healed, and hard-to-heal wounds. For problem skin areas, use a couple drops of frankincense in an equal amount of carrier oil. Frankincense is excellent on mature skin and acne. It is especially good when middle-aged women experience those conditions and also want to prevent wrinkles. Make a compress or massage oil with frankincense for breast cysts or for infection of the lungs, reproductive organs, or urinary tract. It also increases menstrual flow.

GALBANUM

BOTANICAL NAME: *FERULA GALBANIFLUA*

Originating on the slopes of mountain ranges in Iran, galbanum was used in ancient times for incense and perfume. In fact, the biblical book of Exodus mentions galbanum as a component in a sacred incense offering. But the flowering plant's healing and therapeutic properties are even more impressive than its scent. In fact, Hippocrates made use of galbanum with his patients, and the herb was used medicinally in ancient Mesopotamia, India, and China. Often galbanum would be administered in pill form, making it one of the oldest "drugs" in the world.

THERAPEUTIC PROPERTIES

Antispasmodic; improves blood circulation; helps to diminish scars; decongestant; repels insects and parasites.

USED FOR

Galbanum has a relaxing effect on the muscles, and is often used by athletes to treat muscle cramps and pulls. Its ability to improve circulation, especially in the joints, helps to relieve pain from arthritis and rheumatism. Galbanum has been shown to speed up the growth of new cells in scarred areas, making it an ideal remedy for acne scars and stretch marks. When used in incense or sprays, the oil has been shown to repel insects and parasites, including mosquitoes, lice, and bed bugs.

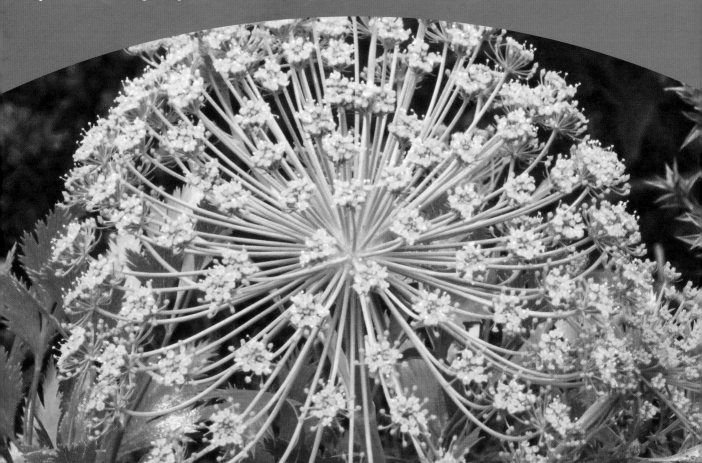

GERANIUM

BOTANICAL NAME: *PELARGONIUM GRAVEOLOENS*

A relative newcomer to the fragrance trade, geranium is a small, tender, South African perennial whose essential oil was not distilled until the nineteenth century. Since it is a veritable medicine cabinet with a lovely scent, it became an instant hit. It is also an insect repellent, and one that is certainly more aromatically pleasing than the commonly used citronella. The scent of geranium mixes well with almost any other essential oil. There are more than 600 varieties, including several with a rose-like fragrance.

THERAPEUTIC PROPERTIES

Antidepressant, antiseptic, astringent; stops bleeding; possibly gently stimulates the adrenals and normalizes hormones.

USED FOR

The essential oil treats a host of problems including inflammation, eczema, acne, burns, infected wounds, fungus (like ringworm), lice, shingles, and herpes. It also decreases scarring and stretch marks. Use it in the form of a salve, cream, lotion, or massage/body oil, whichever is most appropriate. It balances all complexion types and is said to delay wrinkling. Inhale this pleasant scent to treat PMS, menopause, fluid retention, and other hormone-related problems.

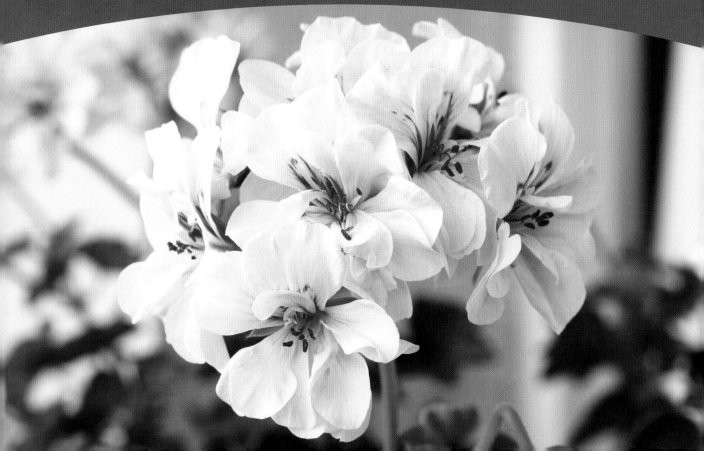

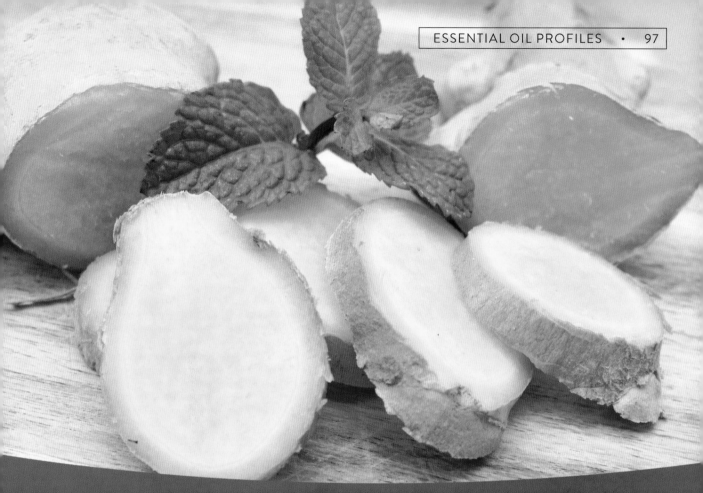

GINGER

BOTANICAL NAME: *ZINGIBER OFFICINALE*

You have certainly encountered ginger's succulent, spicy rhizome in the grocery store. Used fresh, or dried and powdered for a culinary spice, it flavors ginger ale, cakes, and cookies and is a major ingredient in curries and other Eastern cuisines. The Chinese scholar Confucius ate fresh ginger with every meal. Since it was one of the earliest herbs transported in the spice trade, it is now difficult to determine if ginger originated in India or China.

THERAPEUTIC PROPERTIES

Stimulates circulation, increases perspiration, relieves gas and pain, aids digestion.

USED FOR

Use a ginger compress wrapped around the neck or placed on the chest to ease sore throat or lung congestion. The smell of it alone will often open congested sinuses. If you experience nausea or motion sickness, inhale a drop placed on a hankie, eat a little candied ginger, or sip ginger ale, which contains a small amount of the essential oil. To relieve indigestion or menstrual cramps, rub a massage oil containing ginger into the skin on your abdomen or place a poultice made from the grated root on it. In a warming liniment, ginger essential oil treats poor circulation and sore or cramped muscles, since it decreases the substances in the body that make muscles cramp.

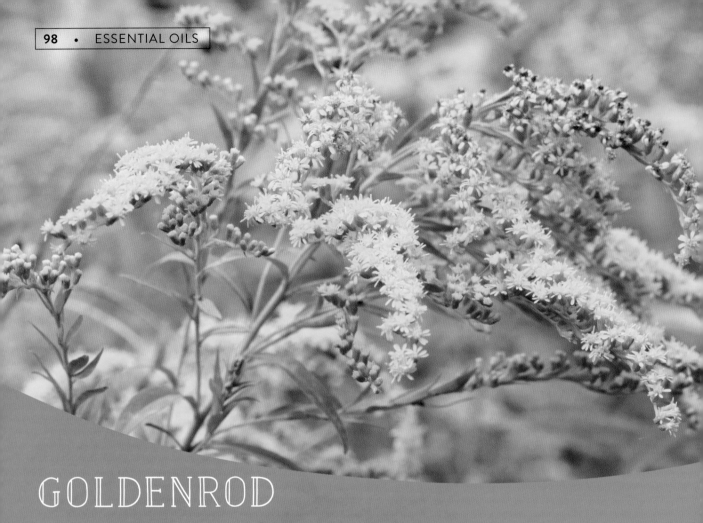

GOLDENROD

BOTANICAL NAME: *SOLIDAGO CANEDENIS*

With their bright yellow flowers and sticky pollen, goldenrods are attractive to bees and butterflies. But the flowers are less attractive to North American gardeners, who often consider the flowers to be weeds. They're also sometimes mistaken for ragweed, and blamed for hay fever allergies, even though goldenrod pollen is too heavy to be carried on the wind. But goldenrods are much more than weeds or a nuisance: the flowers were used in traditional Native American medicine to calm toothaches and sore throats. And Thomas Edison discovered a way to produce rubber from the plants. In fact, Edison's friend Henry Ford gave him a Model T with rubber tires made from goldenrod!

THERAPEUTIC PROPERTIES

Antiseptic and anti-inflammatory; eases cold and allergy symptoms; excellent for use in aromatherapy.

USED FOR

Goldenrod has been shown to help fight urinary tract infections, and its antiseptic and anti-inflammatory properties make it a great choice for treating skin condition like eczema and acne. The oil can help ease congestion and sneezing, whether due to colds or allergies. When used in aromatherapy, goldenrod has an uplifting effect on mood and promotes a sense of calm.

GRAPEFRUIT

BOTANICAL NAME: *CITRUS PARADISI*

Unlike many of the other plants and herbs used for essential oils, grapefruit has a relatively short history. Grapefruits are thought to have naturally occurred sometime after the Indonesian pomelo was introduced to the island of Jamaica in the late 1600s. The fruit was a hybrid between a Jamaican sweet orange and the foreign pomelo, and it became popular throughout the Caribbean. Grapefruit was unknown to the rest of the world until around 1750, when Welsh naturalist Reverend Griffith Hughes made note of it in his book, *The Natural History of Barbados*. Today, not only is the tart, tangy fruit extremely popular, but its essential oil is prized for a host of benefits!

THERAPEUTIC PROPERTIES

Antibacterial; boosts immune system; curbs sugar cravings; natural energizer; excellent oil to use for household cleaners.

USED FOR

Research shows that grapefruit oil is effective at killing many kinds of bacteria, including *E. coli* and salmonella, that can occur on the skin or internally. This also makes it a great choice for fighting acne. Its high vitamin C content naturally boosts the immune system. Inhaling the scent of grapefruit oil, or adding a drop or two to water or tea, has been shown to reduce sugar cravings. The scent is also a sweet-smelling energizer and pick-me-up. Grapefruit oil's uplifting scent and antimicrobial properties make it especially enjoyable to use as household cleaner—it not only kills germs, but it leaves behind a fresh scent!

PRECAUTIONS

Grapefruit oil can negatively interact with some medications, including antidepressants and blood pressure medication. If you take medication, check with a doctor before using the oil. If applied topically, grapefruit can make skin more sensitive to sunlight. After applying, wait at least an hour before heading outdoors, and always use sunscreen.

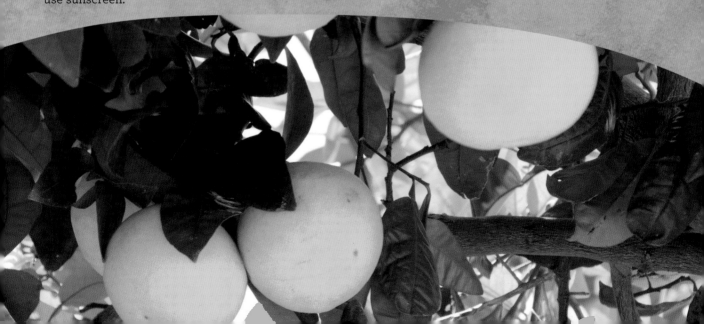

HELICHRYSUM

BOTANICAL NAME: *HELICHRYSUM ITALICUM*

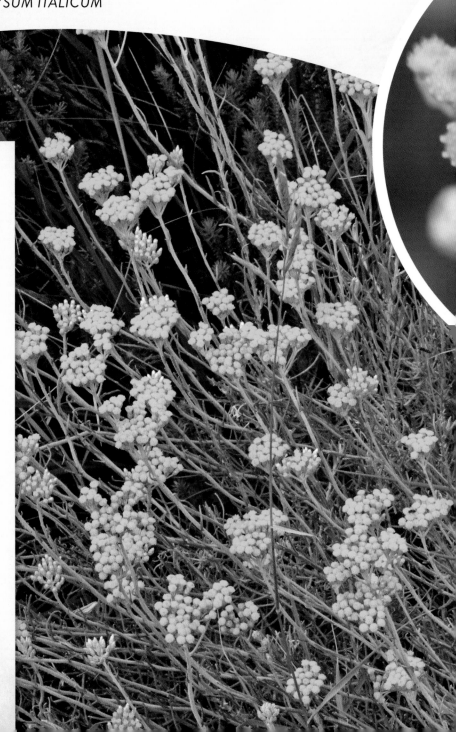

Helichrysum is a small perennial herb. The plant's medicinal and culinary uses go back to the days of ancient Greece. While there are a number of flowering species of helichrysum used in essential oil form, the most commonly available variety is *Helichrysum italicum*. The essential oil is obtained from its clusters of small, golden yellow blossoms.

Helichrysum's aroma is complex but nearly always described as sweet. Think caramelized sugar, honey, and nectar, wrapped in a floral bouquet. Its cloying fragrance is not for everyone, making its aromatherapy applications limited. No matter—this is an oil with amazing regenerative qualities when applied topically. Helichrysum is a skin care superstar: it's ideal for treating scars, blemishes, stretch marks, rashes, acne, and aging skin. It is even effective at treating sprains, muscle pain, and stiffness. Helichrysum promotes the regrowth of skin and the healing of wounds and cuts.

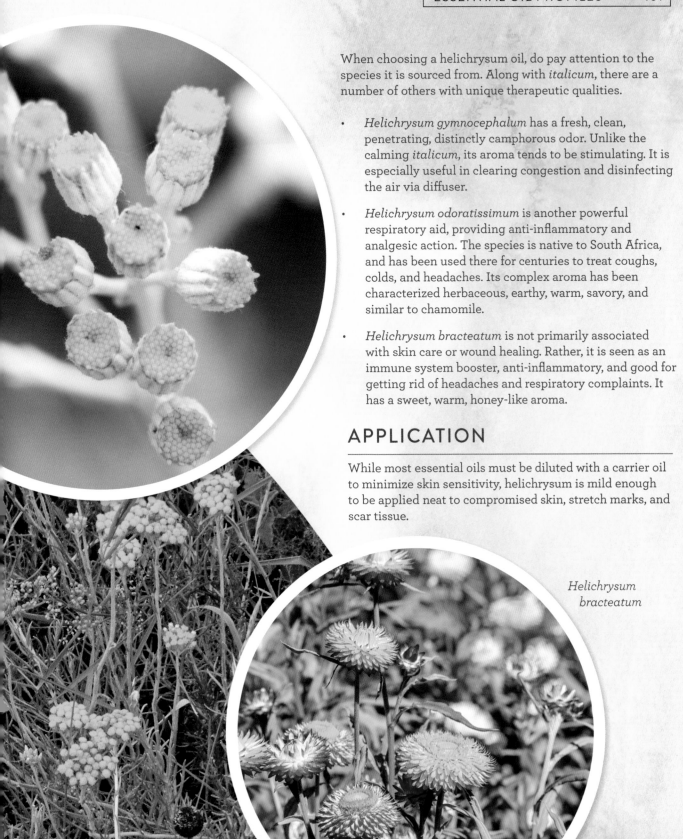

When choosing a helichrysum oil, do pay attention to the species it is sourced from. Along with *italicum*, there are a number of others with unique therapeutic qualities.

- *Helichrysum gymnocephalum* has a fresh, clean, penetrating, distinctly camphorous odor. Unlike the calming *italicum*, its aroma tends to be stimulating. It is especially useful in clearing congestion and disinfecting the air via diffuser.

- *Helichrysum odoratissimum* is another powerful respiratory aid, providing anti-inflammatory and analgesic action. The species is native to South Africa, and has been used there for centuries to treat coughs, colds, and headaches. Its complex aroma has been characterized herbaceous, earthy, warm, savory, and similar to chamomile.

- *Helichrysum bracteatum* is not primarily associated with skin care or wound healing. Rather, it is seen as an immune system booster, anti-inflammatory, and good for getting rid of headaches and respiratory complaints. It has a sweet, warm, honey-like aroma.

APPLICATION

While most essential oils must be diluted with a carrier oil to minimize skin sensitivity, helichrysum is mild enough to be applied neat to compromised skin, stretch marks, and scar tissue.

*Helichrysum
bracteatum*

HINOKI

BOTANICAL NAME: *CHAMAECYPARIS OBTUSA*

The towering hinoki, which can grow to more than 100 feet tall, is a cypress tree native to Japan. The tree is considered an important provider of timber in the country, and it has been used to construct traditional temples, palaces, shrines, and theaters. Because of its strength, appearance, insect-repellent nature, and resistance to rot, hinoki is sometimes called the "divine tree." It's so highly valued in Japan that forests where the tree grows have been protected since the time of the samurai. The wood of the tree has a light lemony scent, and this lovely quality is present in the essential oil, as well.

THERAPEUTIC PROPERTIES

Promotes calm and relaxation; may help with hair growth; natural insect repellent.

USED FOR

Used in a diffuser, the scent of hinoki is calming and helps to relieve anxiety. The oil may help promote hair growth, and is used as an ingredient in many hair products. Just like the wood of the tree, hinoki oil is an insect repellent. Use it to keep unwanted pests out of your home.

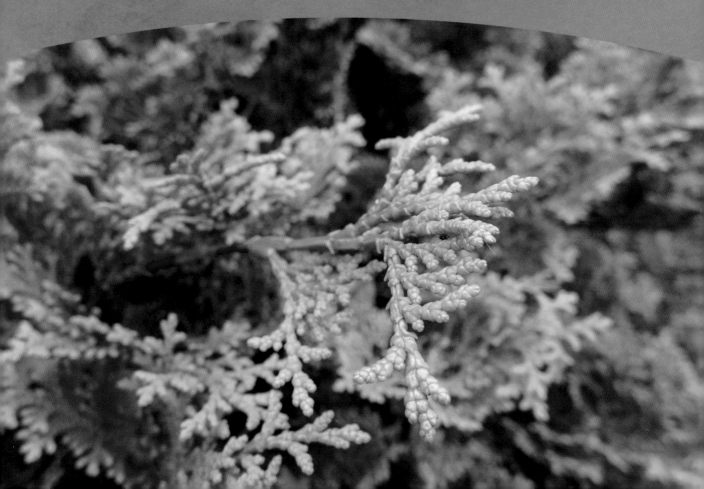

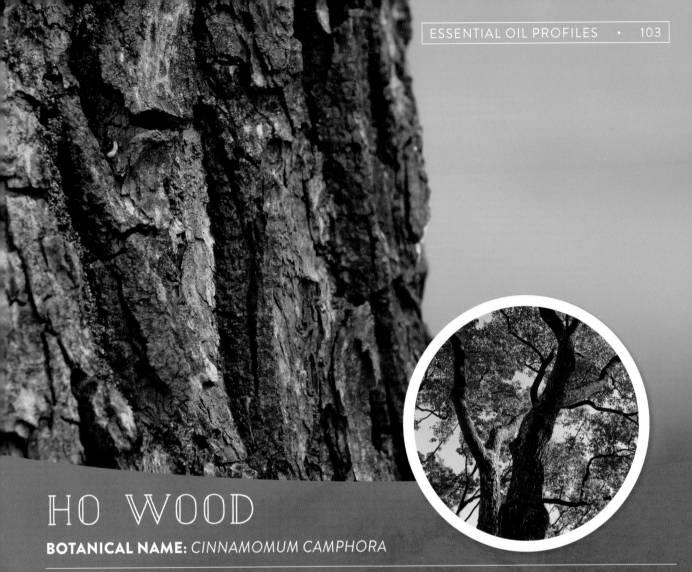

HO WOOD

BOTANICAL NAME: *CINNAMOMUM CAMPHORA*

Ho wood oil is one of the lesser known essential oils on the market. The tree that yields this oil can grow to 100 feet tall and has glossy, waxy leaves that smell of camphor when crushed. But once the wood has been steam distilled, the oil that results has a floral, warm, and slightly sweet aroma that some describe as a mix between tea tree, cinnamon, and lemongrass. Ho wood oil has a high concentration of a substance called linalool, which is known to have antibacterial properties and acts as a natural pest repellent. It's worth checking out this uncommon oil!

THERAPEUTIC PROPERTIES

Antibacterial and anti-inflammatory; reduces stress and anxiety; great for use in skin care; insect repellent.

USED FOR

Ho wood oil can be applied to minor cuts and wounds to prevent infection, while its anti-inflammatory properties reduce swelling and pain. Used in a diffuser, ho wood's calming scent helps to reduce anxiety. The oil encourages new cell growth and has a low comedogenic rating—meaning it won't clog pores. This makes it a useful addition to your skin care routine. Ho wood's high linalool content makes it a natural insect repellent which can ward off mosquitoes, fleas, and cockroaches.

HOLY BASIL

BOTANICAL NAME: *OCIMUM TENUIFLORUM*

Not to be confused with the basil found on a slice of margherita pizza, holy basil is mainly grown for religious and medicinal purposes. The plant—sometimes called tulsi in its native India—is considered a sacred plant in Hinduism. It is grown in many Hindu homes in special pots, and is found next to temples and places of worship. Holy basil has also been used for thousands of years in traditional Ayurvedic medicine, where it is thought to promote longevity and is considered an "elixir of life." And thanks to its essential oil's many healthy benefits, it's not difficult to see why!

THERAPEUTIC PROPERTIES

Antibacterial and antioxidant; good for use in dental care; can help control blood sugar.

USED FOR

Holy basil oil can be used to prevent infections on the skin, and its antibacterial and antioxidant properties make it excellent for use in skin care, to prevent acne and premature aging. The oil can be used in homemade mouthwash, to kill bacteria and freshen breath, and is also an ingredient in some commercial all-natural mouthwashes. Studies have shown that holy basil oil is effective at controlling blood sugar, so it may be useful as a natural diabetes remedy.

PRECAUTIONS

Holy basil oil can be very irritating to the skin, so it should always be diluted in a carrier oil before using. Since it may lower blood sugar, diabetics should consult with a doctor before using.

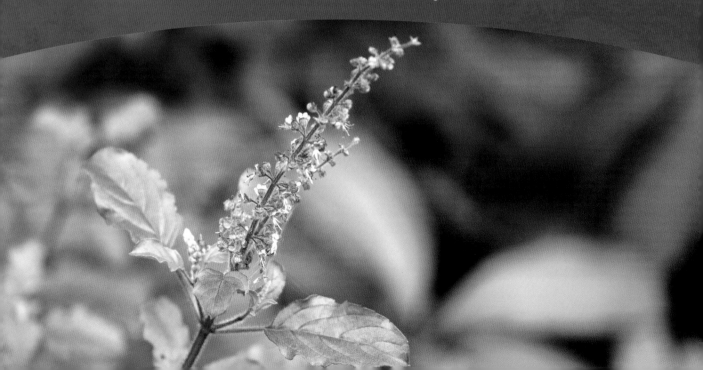

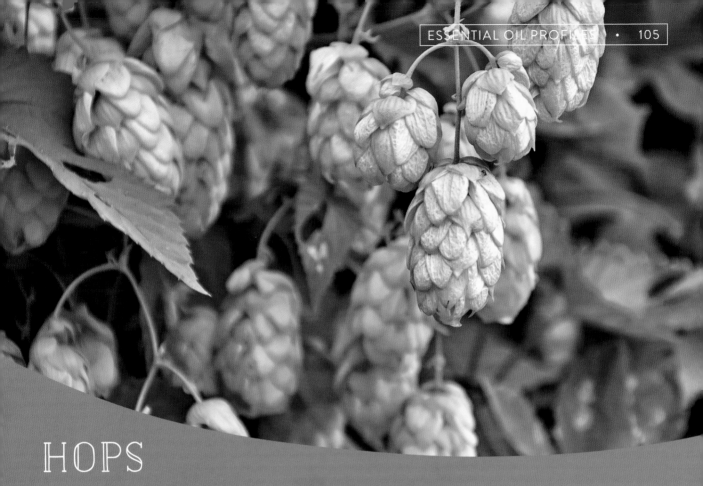

HOPS

BOTANICAL NAME: *HUMULUS LUPULUS*

If you only think of brewing beer when you think of hops, you may be missing out on some great essential oil benefits! The well-known libation ingredient is native to Europe, Asia, and North America, and the fragrant flowers of the plant attract butterflies. The essential oil is derived from these aromatic hops, and the spicy scent is used in perfumes and aromatherapy. Historically, the hops plant has been used as a sedative, and was often placed inside an insomnia sufferer's pillow—which was fittingly called a "hops pillow"—to promote better sleep. Nowadays, the oil can be added to a diffuser or to bath water to produce the same calming effects.

THERAPEUTIC PROPERTIES

Analgesic, anti-inflammatory; helps to relax nervous system.

USED FOR

Hops oil is most popularly used to reduce anxiety, relieve tension headaches, and promote better sleep. The oil has also been shown to relieve chronic pain and to soothe psoriasis and other skin irritations.

PRECAUTIONS

Because of its sedative properties, hops oil can exacerbate symptoms of depression. It is recommended that anyone suffering from depression avoid this essential oil.

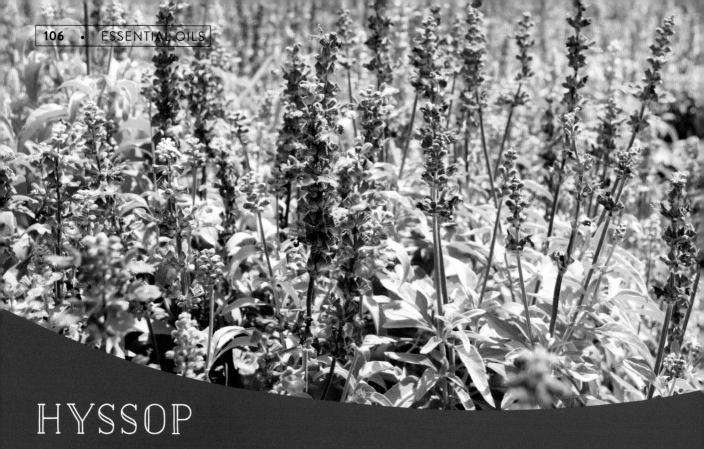

HYSSOP

BOTANICAL NAME: *HYSSOPUS OFFICINALIS*

Hyssop is native to southern Europe and the Middle East, and has been used medicinally since antiquity due to its antiseptic, cough-relieving, and expectorant properties. It was also used for religious purposes in ancient Egypt, where priests would eat the herb during purification rituals. In the Middle Ages, hyssop was used to repel lice, to mask bad smells, and even to ward off plague. And Benedictine monks used the herb to create soups, sauces, and liqueurs. By 1631, the plant had made its way to North America with European settlers, and is now commonly grown throughout the northern United States and Canada. It has a bright medicinal smell that many people will associate with mouthwash.

THERAPEUTIC PROPERTIES

Antiseptic, antiviral, antispasmodic; helps stimulate digestive system; helpful for relieving respiratory ailments.

USED FOR

Hyssop has been shown to prevent infections when applied to wounds, and is effective against viral infections such as colds and flu. Its antispasmodic properties make it a great choice for calming coughs, and hyssop tea can soothe a sore throat. When used in steam inhalation, the oil helps to ease breathing and clear the respiratory tract. Hyssop has also been shown to stimulate the digestive system, and reduce discomfort due to indigestion or gas.

PRECAUTIONS

Hyssop oil contains a compound called pinocamphone, which can stimulate the nerves and cause seizures, especially in people with epilepsy. Those with epilepsy should avoid the oil.

JASMINE

BOTANICAL NAME: *JASMINUM OFFICINALIS* AND *J. GRANDIFLORUM*

The small white flowers of this vinelike evergreen shrub, with their intriguing, complex scent, are intensely fragrant and found in most great perfumes. Jasmine is also known as "mistress of the night" and "moonlight of the grove" because its seductive scent reaches its peak late at night. Even the production of the essential oil is exotic. The flowers are gathered at night, when they produce the most oil, and laid on a layer of fat when using the enfleurage method. Try as chemists might to make it, the scent cannot be duplicated. Synthetic jasmine is so harsh, it demands a touch of the true essential oil to soften it.

THERAPEUTIC PROPERTIES

Antidepressant; relaxes nerves, relieves muscle spasms and cramping.

USED FOR

Jasmine sedates the nervous system, so it is good for jangled nerves, headaches, insomnia, and depression and for taking the emotional edge off PMS and menopause, although keep in mind its age-old reputation as an aphrodisiac! Studies at Toho University School of Medicine in Tokyo show that jasmine also enhances mental alertness and stimulates brain waves. It also eases muscle cramping, such as menstrual cramps. Cosmetically, the oil is wonderful for sensitive or mature skin. In its native India, jasmine flowers infused into sesame oil are applied to abscesses and sores that are difficult to heal. A similar preparation can be made by adding 2 drops of jasmine essential oil to 1 ounce carrier oil.

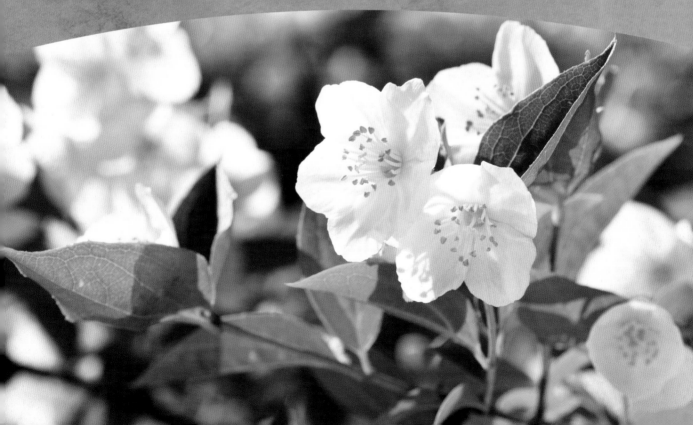

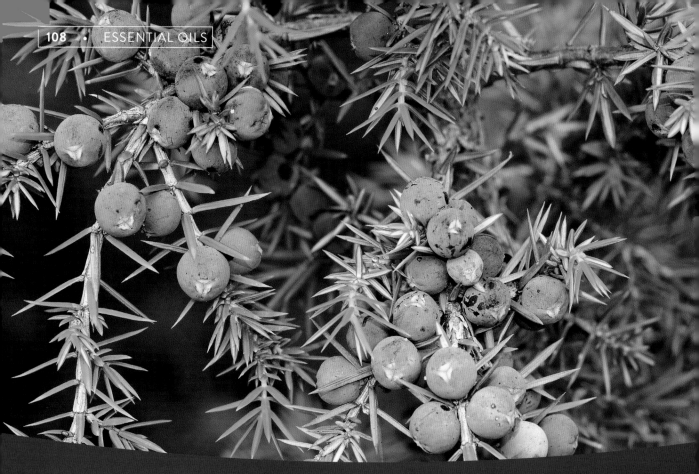

JUNIPER BERRY

BOTANICAL NAME: *JUNIPERUS COMMUNIS*

Burning juniper branches was found to ward off contagious diseases, so medieval physicians chewed the berries while on duty and burned the branches in hospitals. In World War II, the French returned to burning juniper in hospitals as an antiseptic when their supply of drugs ran low. Fresh berries offer the highest quality oil, but needles, branches, and berries that have already been distilled to flavor gin are sometimes used. With many of the same properties as cedarwood, it also acts as a wool moth repellent.

THERAPEUTIC PROPERTIES

Antiseptic, astringent; relieves the aches of rheumatism, arthritis, and sore muscles; increases urination and circulation; encourages menstruation.

USED FOR

Juniper berry essential oil is used in massage oils, liniments, and baths to treat arthritic and rheumatic pain, varicose veins, hemorrhoids, fluid retention (especially before menstruation), and bladder infection. Inhale it in a steam to relieve bronchial congestion, infection, and bronchial spasms. Inhalation may also lift your spirits, as sniffing the oil seems to work as a pick-me-up and to counter general debility. Cosmetically it is suitable for acne complexions and eczema. Add approximately 6 drops per ounce to shampoos for greasy hair or dandruff.

LAVENDER

BOTANICAL NAME: *LAVANDULA ANGUSTIFOLIA*

A well-loved Mediterranean herb, lavender has been associated with cleanliness since Romans first added it to their bathwater. In fact, the name comes from the Latin *lavandus,* meaning to wash. Today lavender remains a favorite for scenting clothing and closets, soaps, and even furniture polish. Lavender was traditionally inhaled to ease exhaustion, insomnia, irritability, and depression. Two related plants called spike (*L. latifolia*) and lavandin (*L. intermedia*) are produced in greater quantities; but they are more camphorous and harsher in scent, with inferior healing properties, although they are useful for disinfecting.

THERAPEUTIC PROPERTIES

Antiseptic, circulatory stimulant; relieves muscle spasms and cramping.

USED FOR

Lavender is among the safest and most widely used of all aromatherapy oils. It relieves muscle pain, migraines and other headaches, and inflammation. It is also one of the most antiseptic essential oils, treating many types of infection, including lung, sinus, and vaginal infections. Lavender is suitable for all skin types. Cosmetically, it appears to be a cell regenerator. It prevents scarring and stretch marks and reputedly slows the development of wrinkles. It is used on burns, sun-damaged skin, wounds, rashes, and, of course, skin infections. Of several fragrances tested by aromatherapy researchers, lavender was most effective at relaxing brain waves and reducing stress.

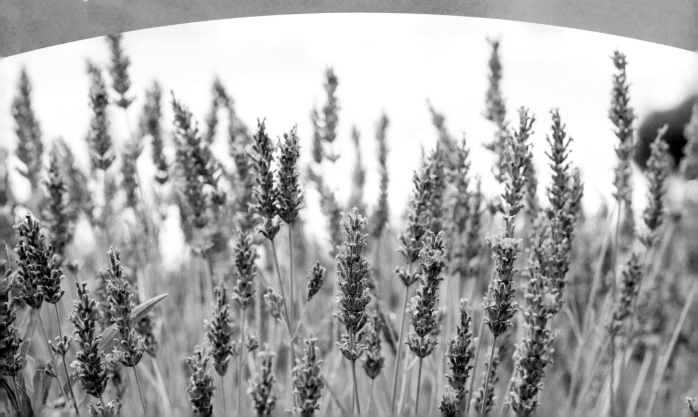

LEMON

BOTANICAL NAME: *CITRUS LIMONUM*

Most people would describe lemon as having a "clean" smelling fragrance. Aromatherapists use the tie-in with cleanliness to help people purge feelings of imperfection and impurity and to build up their confidence. Lemon essential oil is a major ingredient in commercial beverages, foods, and pharmaceuticals, although the cheaper lemongrass or even synthetic citral is often added to stretch it. It also is popular for its fresh aroma in cologne and many cosmetics, especially cleansing creams and lotions.

The flowers are occasionally distilled for their pleasant aroma, but cold pressing the peel produces the essential oil that you are most likely to find. Like other citruses, the oil keeps well for only about a year; so you can prolong its life by storing it in a cool place or even in the refrigerator.

THERAPEUTIC PROPERTIES

Antiseptic, antidepressant, antiviral; decreases indigestion, stops bleeding.

USED FOR

Studies show that the oil increases the activity of the immune system by stimulating the production of the white corpuscles that fight infection. Additionally, lemon essential oil counters a wide range of viral and bacterial infections. Massage it on the skin in a carrier oil base to relieve congested lymph glands. Inhaled it has been shown to reduce blood pressure. Since it also reduces water retention and increases mineral absorption, it can be helpful in achieving weight loss. Incorporated into cosmetics, lemon is best used on oily complexions and to clean acne, blackheads, and other skin impurities.

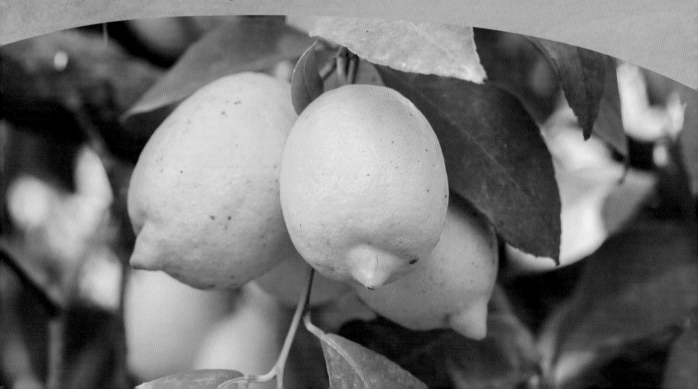

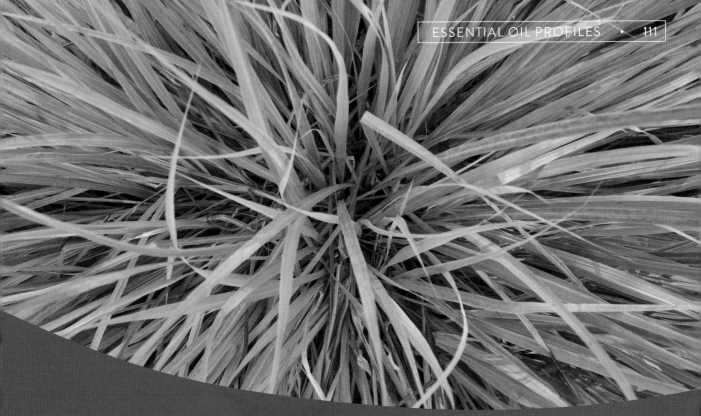

LEMONGRASS

BOTANICAL NAME: *CYMBOPOGON CITRATUS*

A relatively inexpensive essential oil, lemongrass is often the source of the lemon scent found in cosmetics and hair preparations. Its pleasant, clean fragrance is also incorporated into soaps, perfumes, and deodorants, and it flavors many canned and frozen foods. No wonder it is one of the ten best-selling essential oils in the world.

Along with related oils such as the lemon-rose scented palmarosa (*C. martini*) and citronella (*C. nardus*), it often adulterates more costly essential oils like melissa and lemon verbena to stretch quantities. Palmarosa is frequently used in skin preparations, while citronella is well known as an insect repellent and cleanser. The yellow to amber oil of these grasses is distilled from their partially dried leaves.

THERAPEUTIC PROPERTIES

Antiseptic, deodorant, astringent; relieves rheumatic and other pain, relaxes nerves.

USED FOR

Researchers also found this refreshing fragrance to reduce headaches and irritability and to prevent drowsiness. To make a foot bath, add about 3 drops of lemongrass oil to 2 or 3 quarts of warm water in a small tub. Stir well and keep your feet in the water for at least 20 minutes. You can also add a few drops to your bath. Lemongrass is an antiseptic suitable for use on various types of skin infections, usually as a wash or compress, and is especially effective on ringworm and infected sores. In fact, studies found that it is more effective against staph infection than either penicillin or streptomycin. When sprayed on a counter top, or along walls and floors, it discourages insect invasions and mold.

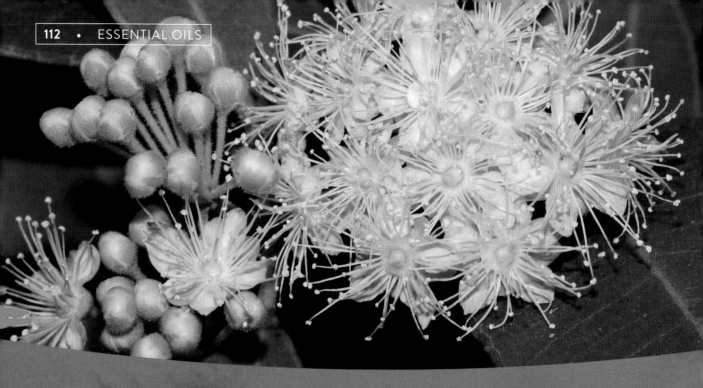

LEMON MYRTLE

BOTANICAL NAME: *BACKHOUSIA CITRIODORA*

Named after English botanist James Backhouse, *Backhousia citriodora* was once commonly known as lemon-scented myrtle. Eventually, the name was shortened to "lemon myrtle," to help the edible herb achieve more popularity in the culinary world. The lemony dried leaves are used in everything from sweet desserts to savory pastas, and are also popular in soaps, lotions, and bath products. The plant is native to Australia, where indigenous people have used it for medicine for hundreds of years due to its antimicrobial properties. Even today, the majority of lemon myrtle used for essential oil is grown only in Queensland and New South Wales, Australia.

THERAPEUTIC PROPERTIES

Antimicrobial, antifungal, anti-inflammatory; helps to relieve anxiety and stress; deodorizes; used in bath products.

USED FOR

Lemon myrtle's antimicrobial properties make it ideal for treating skin conditions such as acne and psoriasis, or preventing infections in minor cuts and scrapes. It can also ease itching and inflammation caused by insect bites and stings. It may help boost the immune system and keep colds and flu at bay. A few drops in bathwater help to relax the mind as well as the muscles. Lemon myrtle makes an excellent cleaner for your home, thanks to its antiseptic qualities and uplifting scent.

PRECAUTIONS

Because of its citric quality, lemon myrtle may make skin more susceptible to sunburn. If used topically, avoid direct exposure to sunlight for 48 hours.

LIME

BOTANICAL NAME: *CITRUS AURANTIFOLIA*

Lime trees may be best known for providing the crucial ingredient in delicious key lime pies, but the tree is beneficial for more than just your taste buds. Lime has been used for therapeutic purposes since prehistoric times, when the leaves of the tree were used to treat bug bites and injuries. In the 19th century, British sailors would use the vitamin C rich fruit to prevent scurvy and skin problems. In fact, it is said that the sailor nickname "limey" came about because of the fruit's popularity with sailors! Today, lime oil is widely used in the food and beverage industry due to its refreshing, tart taste, but the same antioxidant properties that protected sailors still provide us with healthy benefits today.

THERAPEUTIC PROPERTIES

Antibacterial, antiviral, astringent; helps to stop bleeding from fresh wounds; excellent for use in aromatherapy.

USED FOR

Lime oil has been shown to protect against infections in minor cuts and scrapes, as well as ward off colds and flu. It works well to heal skin conditions such as psoriasis, rashes, and acne. Its astringent properties can help tone and tighten skin, keep gums healthy, and stop bleeding from minor injuries. Use a few drops in a diffuser for an uplifting, energizing scent.

PRECAUTIONS

As with other citrus-based oils, lime oil may make skin more susceptible to sunburn. If used topically, avoid direct exposure to sunlight for 48 hours.

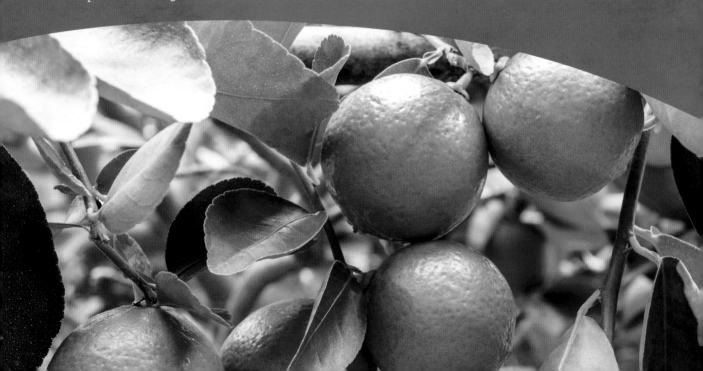

LITSEA CUBEBA

BOTANICAL NAME: *LITSEA CUBEBA*

Also known as aromatic litsea and may chang, litsea cubeba is an evergreen tree native to Southeast Asia. The tree bears a fruit that resembles a pepper, giving it the nickname "mountain pepper." The essential oil—which has a lemony, citrusy scent similar to lemongrass—is extracted from these ripened and dried pepper-like fruits. The oil has traditionally been used in Chinese medicine to help with digestive issues, muscle aches, and asthma, and to relieve stress and anxiety. Although litsea cubeba is one of the least common essential oils on the market, its benefits should convince you to give it a try!

THERAPEUTIC PROPERTIES

Antibacterial, antiviral, antifungal, anti-inflammatory; helps reduce stress and anxiety; used to relieve digestive upset; insect repellent and home cleaner.

USED FOR

Effective in killing bacteria, viruses, and fungi, litsea cubeba aids a host of problems, including acne, athlete's foot, insect bites, and ringworm. The uplifting scent has been used for hundreds of years in aromatherapy to induce feelings of calm and reduce stress. A few drops added to a carrier oil and massaged into your stomach can reduce indigestion and stomach upset. The oil makes a great cleaner for your home, and the fresh-smelling scent helps keep bugs at bay.

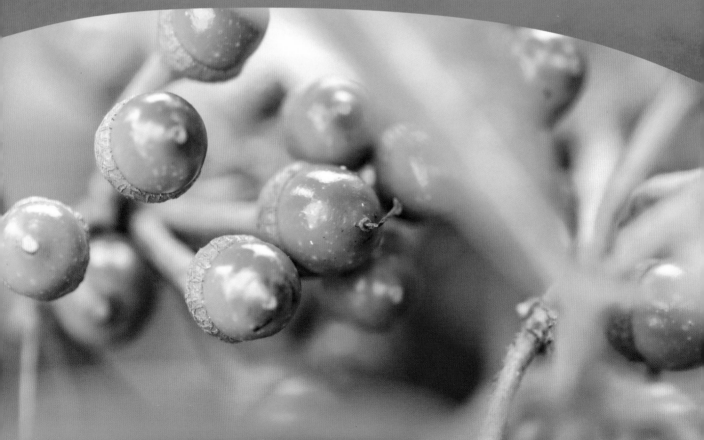

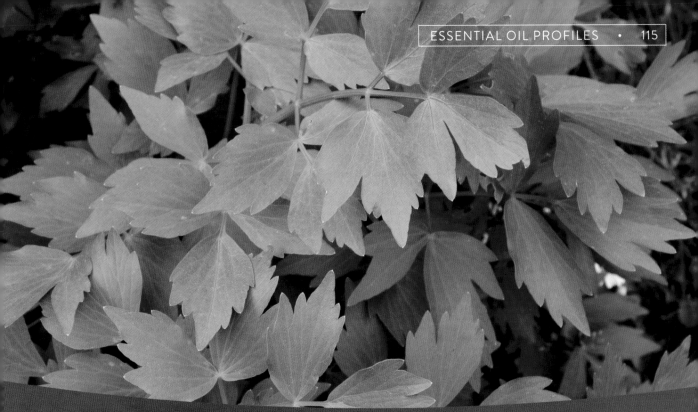

LOVAGE

BOTANICAL NAME: *LEVISTICUM OFFICINALE*

The origins of lovage, a robust plant that grows to more than eight feet tall, are disputed. But the perennial has been extensively cultivated for hundreds of years in southern Europe as a culinary herb and vegetable. Its flavor is described as a mix between celery and parsley. Some say the Romans were the first to use the plant for medicinal purposes, using it to reduce fever and treat stomach upset. In the Middle Ages, the herb was a popular treatment for malaria, sore throats, and kidney stones. Although all parts of the plant have historically been used medicinally, it is usually the roots that are steam distilled to produce the essential oil.

THERAPEUTIC PROPERTIES

Anti-inflammatory; helps treat allergies; skin soothing; eases digestion.

USED FOR

Lovage's anti-inflammatory properties make it helpful for relieving symptoms of arthritis or gout. The oil is a natural inhibitor of histamine, which can reduce allergic responses in the body. Lovage is soothing to the skin and can be used to treat conditions like psoriasis and acne. The oil may help relieve upset stomachs and relieve bloating and gas.

PRECAUTIONS

Lovage oil is known to cause photosensitivity. If applied to the skin, avoid sunlight for 48 hours, or make sure it is diluted to less than one percent.

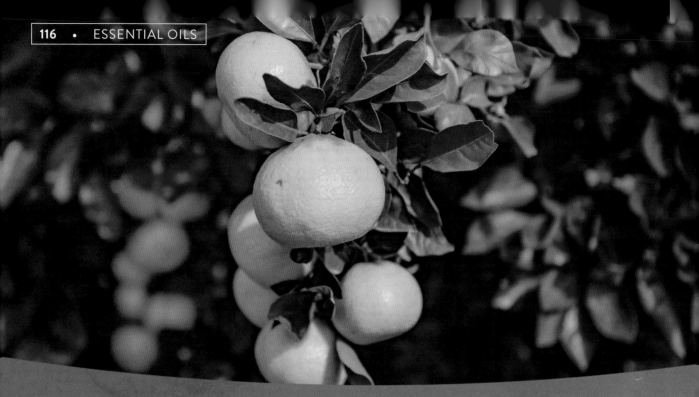

MANDARIN

BOTANICAL NAME: *CITRUS RETICULATA*

If you've ever received a mandarin orange in your Christmas stocking, you may have the Japanese to thank. The sweet citrus fruit has traditionally been given as a gift for the New Year in the Asian country. And in the 1880s, when Japanese immigrants in the United States would receive boxes of mandarins from their families at the New Year, the rest of the country began to take notice. Soon the tradition spread across the U.S., and special "Orange Trains" carried the fruit across the country after the November harvest. Eventually, the sight of mandarins was a sign that the holidays were officially approaching. Fortunately, you don't need to wait for a holiday to enjoy the benefits of mandarin essential oil!

THERAPEUTIC PROPERTIES

Antimicrobial; useful in skin care: reduces stress and anxiety; excellent as a household cleanser.

USED FOR

Mandarin oil protects wounds from infection, and is also especially good at protecting food from bacterial growth. It helps to prevent acne and diminishes the appearance of stretch marks and scars. The uplifting scent of mandarin helps relieve stress and anxiety, and even quells nausea. Thanks to its antimicrobial properties and great scent, the oil is perfect to use as a natural household cleaner and air freshener.

PRECAUTIONS

Like many citrus oils, mandarin can cause phototoxicity. If applied to the skin, stay out of direct sunlight for 48 hours.

MANUKA

BOTANICAL NAME: *LEPTOSPERMUM SCOPARIUM*

Although the manuka tree is sometimes called "tea tree," manuka oil is not the same as tea tree oil. The manuka, which is native to Australia and New Zealand, was dubbed "tea tree" by famed British explorer Captain James Cook. Captain Cook would use the leaves of the manuka tree to brew tea (and also beer!). But long before Captain Cook, the Maori in New Zealand were using manuka to cure fevers, treat colds, and soothe aching muscles. Today, manuka oil can be found in a myriad of skin care products on the market, but the pure essential oil is prized for a host of other benefits!

THERAPEUTIC PROPERTIES

Antibacterial, antifungal, and anti-inflammatory; great for skin care and hair care; promotes new cell growth.

USED FOR

Manuka oil has been shown to be very effective against bacteria, making it a great oil to use for cuts, scrapes, and bug bites. There's good reason it's included in so many skin care products: the oil's antibacterial, antifungal, and anti-inflammatory properties help keep skin clear, keep dandruff at bay, and calm irritation. And manuka encourages new cell growth, helping scars and stretch marks fade.

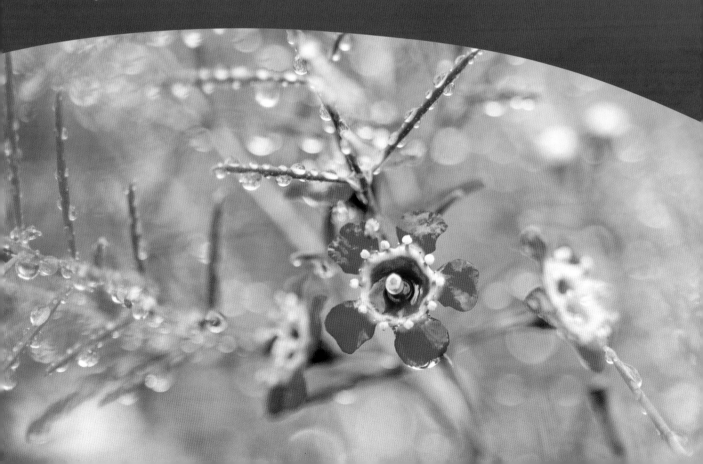

MARJORAM

BOTANICAL NAME: *ORIGANUM MARJORANA*

The greenish-yellow oil is distilled from the plant's flowering tops. Its taste and properties are milder than the closely related oregano, which is so strong and potentially toxic that it is seldom used in aromatherapy. The odor is sweet, herby, and pungent in concentration. When diluted, it mellows to an almost warm, spicy floral with a hint of camphor.

THERAPEUTIC PROPERTIES

Antioxidant; calms nerves, clears mucous from the lungs, relieves pain, improves digestion, brings on menstruation, lowers high blood pressure, stops bleeding.

USED FOR

A good sedative, marjoram eases stiff joints and muscle spasms, including tics, excessive coughing, menstrual cramps, and headaches (especially migraines). It also slightly lowers high blood pressure. Testing has shown it to be one of the most effective fragrances in relaxing brain waves. As a result, it makes an excellent calming massage oil, delightful when combined with the softer lavender. Add a few drops to your bath to counter stress or insomnia. Since it has specific properties that fight the viruses and bacteria responsible for colds, flu, or laryngitis, add a few drops of essential oil to either a chest balm or bath, or put 2 or 3 drops in a bowl of hot water and inhale the steam. In healing salves and creams, it also soothes burns, bruises, and inflammation. Marjoram is also an antioxidant that naturally preserves food.

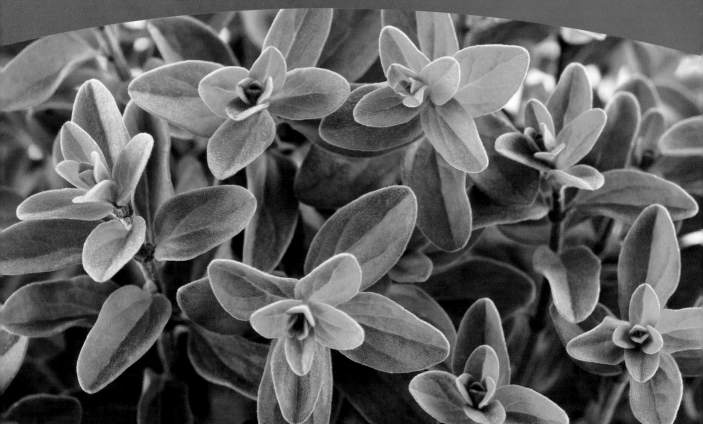

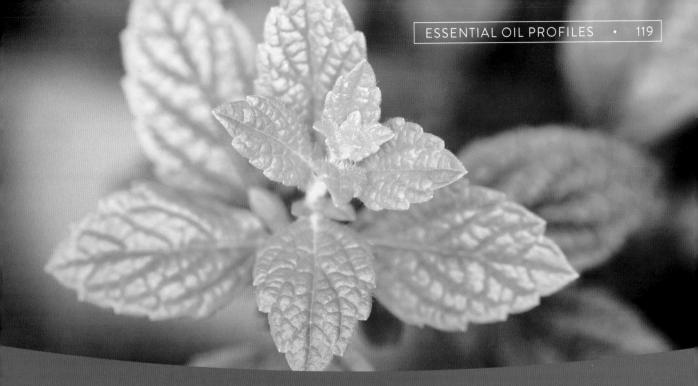

MELISSA

BOTANICAL NAME: *MELISSA OFFICINALIS*

Melissa, which is often referred to as lemon balm, is native to Europe and central Asia. The perennial plant produces small white flowers in the summertime that are full of nectar, making melissa useful for attracting bees for honey production. In fact, *melissa* is the Greek word for the honeybee. Melissa essential oil tends to be more expensive than many other oils on the market, but this is for good reason: it takes between 3.5 and 7.5 tons of plant material to produce just one pound of the essential oil! If you find a cheap bottle of melissa oil, chances are it's been mixed with lemongrass or citronella. But with all of melissa's amazing benefits, it may be worth it to splurge on the pure stuff!

THERAPEUTIC PROPERTIES

Antibiotic, antiviral, and anti-inflammatory; may help control blood sugar; lifts mood; helps lower blood pressure.

USED FOR

Melissa oil's antibiotic, antiviral, and anti-inflammatory properties make it an excellent choice for all kinds of skin care. It can protect wounds from infection, calm eczema and acne, and has even been shown to kill the herpes virus that causes cold sores. Studies have shown that melissa improves blood glucose levels and triglyceride levels, and helps to lower cholesterol. When used in a diffuser, the lemony scent quells stress and anxiety, promoting calm and lowering blood pressure.

PRECAUTIONS

Those with hypothyroidism should avoid using melissa oil, as it can block the absorption of thyroid medication.

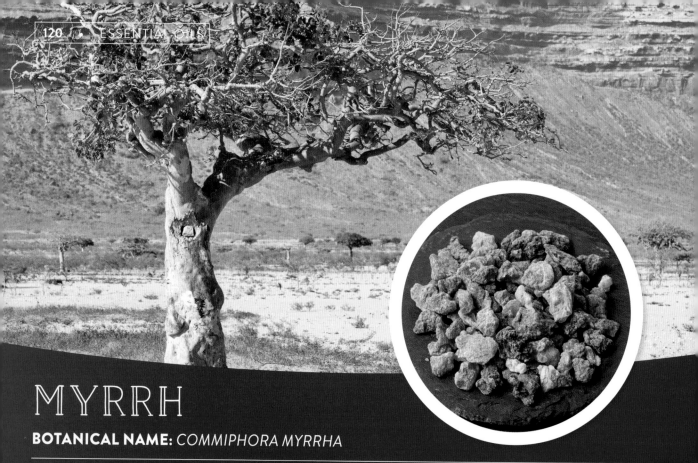

MYRRH

BOTANICAL NAME: *COMMIPHORA MYRRHA*

This small, scrubby, spiny tree from the Middle East and North East Africa is not very handsome, but it makes up for its looks with the precious gum it exudes. An important trade item for several thousand years, myrrh was a primary ingredient in ancient cosmetics and incenses. Believed to comfort sorrow, its name means "bitter tears." This may also refer to the bitter-tasting myrrh sap, which oozes in drops when the tree's bark is cut. Myrrh was added to wine by both the Greeks and Hebrews to heighten sensual awareness. The yellow to amber-colored oil is distilled from the gum and frequently added to toothpastes and gum preparations to help alleviate mouth ulcers, gum inflammation, and infection.

THERAPEUTIC PROPERTIES

Antiseptic, anti-inflammatory, antibacterial, antifungal, decongestant, astringent; heals wounds, brings on menstruation.

USED FOR

Myrrh is an expensive but effective treatment for chapped, cracked, or aged skin, eczema, bruises, infection, varicose veins, ringworm, and athlete's foot. Included in many ointments, it dries weepy wounds. It is a specific remedy for mouth and gum disease and is found in many oral preparations. It is very helpful applied on herpes sores and blisters: Add it to a lip balm, using about 25 drops per ounce. Lozenges or syrup containing myrrh treat coughs. As an additional bonus, it increases the activity of the immune system.

PRECAUTIONS

Due to a possible increase of thyroid activity, do not use myrrh if you have an overactive thyroid.

MYRTLE

BOTANICAL NAME: *MYRTUS COMMUNIS*

A flowering evergreen shrub, myrtle originated in Africa and southern Europe. According to Greek mythology, the plant was sacred to the goddesses Aphrodite and Demeter, and the plant is mentioned numerous times in ancient Greek and Roman writings. Myrtle has a long history of medicinal use, having been prescribed for fever and pain relief since at least 2500 BC. This may be due to its high concentration of salicylic acid, which is a compound related to aspirin and other modern-day pain relievers. Myrtle's scent is similar to eucalyptus oil, and, in fact, it comes from the same family as both eucalyptus and tea tree.

THERAPEUTIC PROPERTIES

Antimicrobial, antiseptic, anti-inflammatory; decongestant and expectorant; deodorant.

USED FOR

Myrtle oil can be applied to cuts and scrapes to prevent infection, or used to address skin conditions like acne. When used in a diffuser, the oil can help relieve congestion, coughs, and bronchial infections. Myrtle also makes an excellent deodorizer, either when used as incense or applied to the body like deodorant.

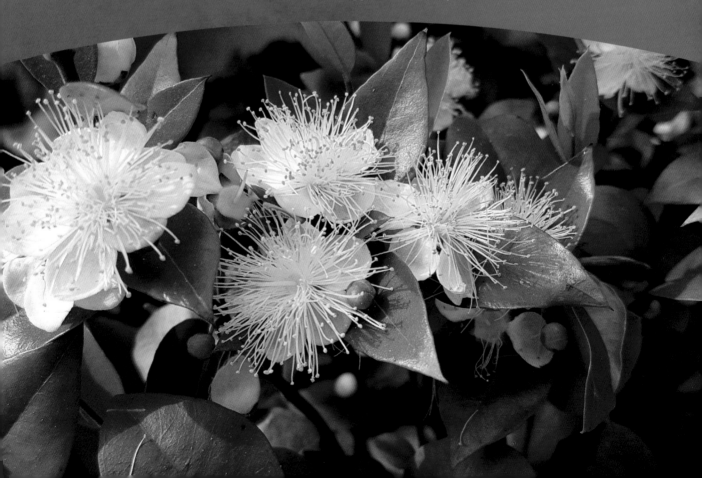

NEROLI

BOTANICAL NAME: *CITRUS AURANTIUM*

An Indochina native, the bitter orange produces the blossoms used for an oil known to aromatherapists and perfumers as neroli. Modern aromatherapists regard neroli as a treatment for depression. The blossoms may be distilled, made into a concrete by enfleurage, or extracted with solvents to create an absolute. A by-product of distillation, "orange flower water," is used in cooking and as a skin toner. Neroli is the main ingredient of the original eau de cologne, which was used both as a body fragrance and as a skin toner. Distilling the leaves and stems of the bitter orange produces an essential oil called petitgrain that is frequently used in men's cologne today and often adulterates the far more expensive neroli.

THERAPEUTIC PROPERTIES

Sedative; relieves muscle spasms and cramping, stimulates circulation.

USED FOR

Neroli's favored use is for circulation problems, especially hemorrhoids and high blood pressure. It makes a wonderfully fragrant and effective cosmetic for mature, dry, and sensitive skin and is also one of the best essential oils to add to a vaginal cream during menopause. It reputedly regenerates skin cells and has anti-aging properties. For the ultimate luxury, add it to your bath to ease tension from PMS, menopause, or life in general.

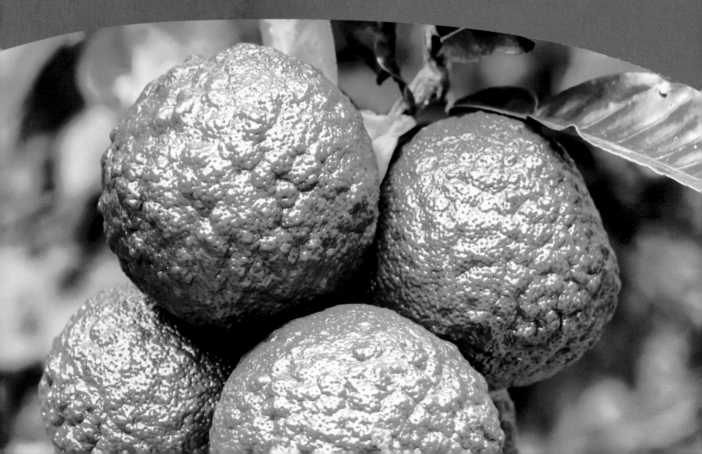

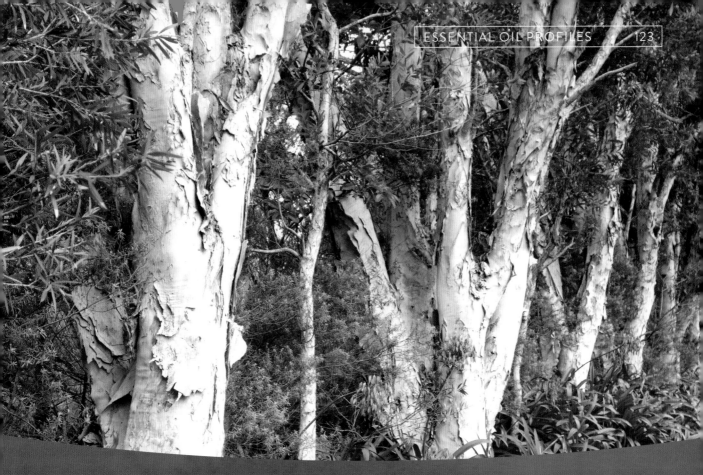

NIAOULI

BOTANICAL NAME: *MELALEUCA QUINQUENERVIA*

Native to Papua New Guinea and the eastern Australian coast, the niaouli tree is commonly known as the broad-leaved paperbark or the paperbark tea tree. The tree has long been popular in Australia, where indigenous peoples have prized it for hundreds of years thanks to its many uses. Indigenous Australians found the crushed leaves to be soothing for colds and headaches, and also used its thick, papery bark to line ground ovens and construct cooking utensils and shelter. The tree was introduced to the United States sometime in the 1900s, and is now considered a destructive, invasive species in many states. Fortunately, niaouli essential oil is anything but destructive!

THERAPEUTIC PROPERTIES

Antibacterial; analgesic; great for treating cold and flu symptoms.

USED FOR

Although similar to tea tree oil, niaouli is gentler on the skin and less likely to cause irritation. This makes it an excellent choice for preventing skin infections in cuts, scrapes, and insect bites. The oil works well as an analgesic, reducing muscle aches and pain from headaches and toothaches. Used in a diffuser, niaouli helps to ease congestion and coughs due to colds and flu.

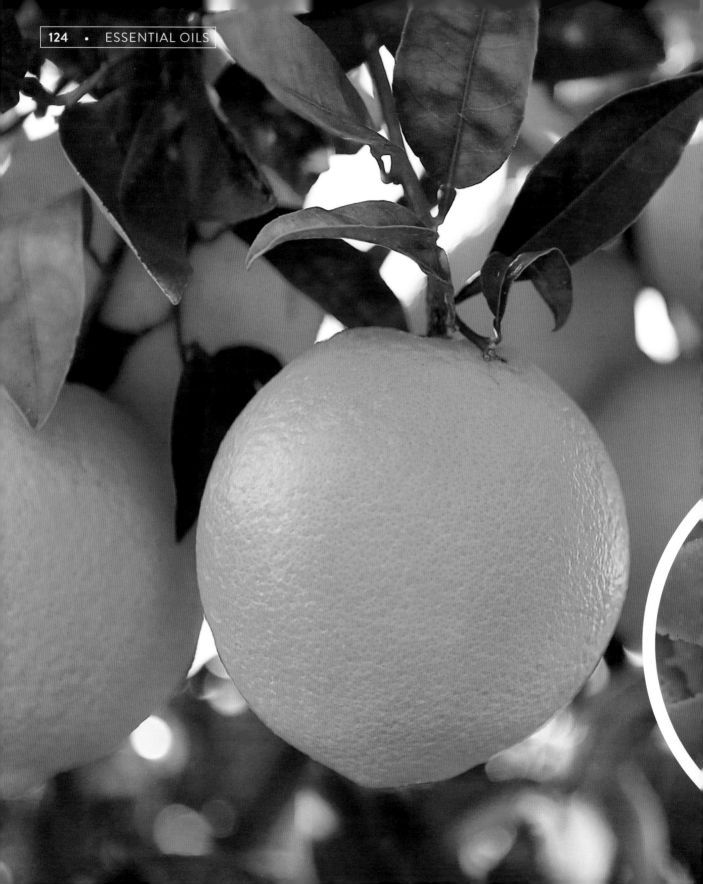

ORANGE

BOTANICAL NAME: *CITRUS SINENSIS*

Dispersed throughout the Mediterranean during the time of the crusades, the familiar sweet orange now comes from Sicily, Israel, Spain, and the U.S., each country's essential oil offering slightly different characteristics. They are rich in vitamins A, B, and C, flavonoids, and minerals. The Chinese, however, correctly warned in the *Chu-lu*—the first monograph describing the various citruses that was written in 1178—that they can increase lung congestion.

Oranges were considered symbols of fruitfulness, and the Greeks called them the "golden apple of the Hesperides." The god Zeus is said to have given an orange to his bride Hera at their wedding.

In 1290, Eleanor of Castile brought oranges to England, where they were grown as luxuries in greenhouses or "orangeries." In northern climates, only the very wealthy could afford oranges, and they were often given as extravagant gifts at Christmas time. In European courts they were stuck with cloves and carried as a pomander to dispel disagreeable odors and emotions such as depression and nervousness, as well as to bring more cheer into dreary winter days. The essential oil is cold pressed from the peel and lasts only about a year, so keep it cool and away from direct sunlight.

Orange's greatest claim to aromatherapy fame is its ability to affect moods and to lower high blood pressure. In fact, just sniffing it lowers blood pressure a couple points. It is also a good adjunct treatment for irregular heartbeat. Research at International Flavors and Fragrances, Inc., in New Jersey found that orange also reduces anxiety. You don't even need to buy the essential oil; simply peel an orange and inhale its aroma. Although not as antibiotic as lemon, it still has some value in fighting flu, colds, and breaking up congested lymph, especially when added to massage oil. The aroma of oranges is a favorite of children, and they will usually be more enthusiastic about an aromatherapy treatment when it is included. Also use the massage oil to ease a bout of indigestion or overcome a light case of insomnia or depression. Cosmetically it is good for oily complexions, although essential oils with more sophisticated fragrances are preferred.

PRECAUTIONS

The oil is only slightly photosensitizing, but still go easy in baths or any skin preparations since it can burn the skin—just 4 drops in a bathtub can be enough to irritate and redden sensitive skin. Related oils such as that of tangerine or mandarin are milder and safer choices for pregnant women and very young children.

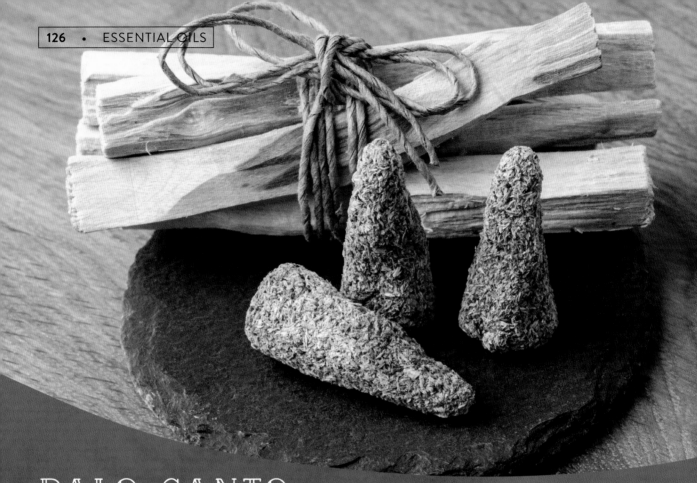

PALO SANTO

BOTANICAL NAME: *BURSERA GRAVEOLENS*

Palo santo, Spanish for "holy wood," is a tree native to Mexico, Central and South America, and the Galapagos Islands. The tree is from the same botanical family as frankincense and myrrh, which are also known for their beneficial essential oils. The oil from the palo santo tree has been used for centuries in folk medicine, as a way to relieve stomachaches and pain from arthritis, and was often burned by medicine men as a way to drive out "bad energy." Today, palo santo is seen as a promising aid for fighting inflammation and boosting immunity. Interestingly, the oil is distilled from fallen branches and dead trees, as palo santo wood develops a unique chemistry once it is dead.

THERAPEUTIC PROPERTIES

Antibacterial, anti-inflammatory; fights colds and flu; bug repellent; excellent household cleaner.

USED FOR

Palo santo's anti-inflammatory properties help to boost the immune system during times of stress or illness, and provide relief from headaches. Add a few drops to a bath to help fight colds and flu. The oil can be combined with water and sprayed on skin or clothes as a natural bug repellent. Its sweet scent and antibacterial effect make it a great choice for disinfecting and deodorizing your home.

PALMAROSA

BOTANICAL NAME: *CYMBOPOGON MARTINII*

Native to India, palmarosa is a species of grass that is often cultivated specifically for its aromatic, sweet, rose-scented oil. In fact, it was given the name "palmarosa"—which means "palm rose"—thanks to its lovely scent. Traditionally, the oil was used to keep insects away from stores of grains and beans, and for treating infections and aches and pains. The leaves were crushed and made into poultices, and the grass and roots were steeped into tea and taken for bronchitis, fevers, and jaundice. Today, palmarosa is mostly used in the perfume and cosmetic industry, but this oil is especially prized for its skin-loving properties.

THERAPEUTIC PROPERTIES

Antibacterial and antiviral; promotes skin hydration and new cell growth; aids digestion; used in soaps and cosmetics.

USED FOR

Palmarosa has been shown to inhibit the growth of bacteria and viruses, making it effective at preventing infection. The oil is excellent for skin care, increasing hydration in the skin and promoting cell growth, and is useful for treating conditions like eczema and psoriasis. The oil helps to increase stomach acid, which aids healthy digestion. Palmarosa's aromatic scent makes it a perfect choice for soaps, lotions, and cosmetics.

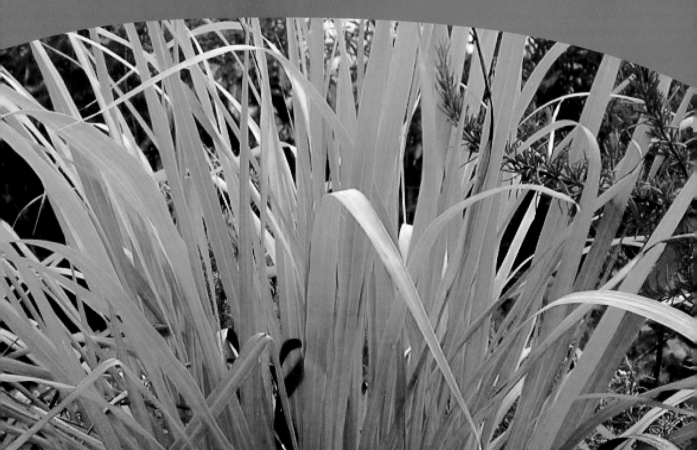

PARSLEY SEED

BOTANICAL NAME: *PETROSELINUM SATIVUM*

Most of us are familiar with parsley as a leafy garnish on restaurant plates, but the Mediterranean herb has been prized for thousands of years for its medicinal benefits, as well as its culinary value. In fact, parsley is one of the oldest spices—and possibly medicines—known to man! Ancient Egyptians and Greeks were familiar with the plant, and the epic poet Homer even mentioned it in the *Odyssey*. Early Greek and Roman physicians found the herb useful for treating kidney and bladder disorders, digestive issues, gallstones, and dysentery. Oil can be extracted from the entire plant, but the seeds contain the highest concentration of this amazing substance.

THERAPEUTIC PROPERTIES

Antimicrobial, diuretic; aids digestion.

USED FOR

Parsley can prevent infections thanks to its antimicrobial properties. As a diuretic, it helps to detoxify the body of unwanted water, salt, and uric acid. This can not only lower blood pressure, but can relieve the symptoms of gout and arthritis, as well. One of parsley's oldest uses was aiding digestive issues, and this is still a great way to use it today: it stimulates digestion, while relieving constipation, indigestion, and gas.

PRECAUTIONS

Parsley seed oil should not be used by pregnant women as it can cause miscarriage.

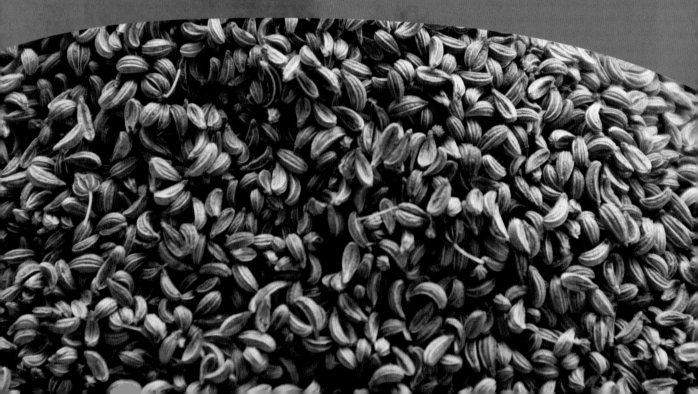

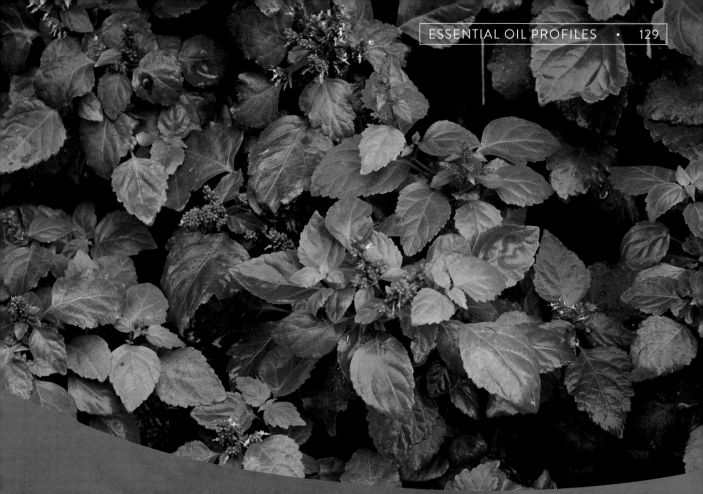

PATCHOULI

BOTANICAL NAME: *POGOSTEMON CABLIN*

To some people the scent of patchouli is exotic, sensual, and luxurious, but to others it's too forceful and repellent. It is so overpowering that most cosmetics forgo its virtues in favor of other essential oils that are more universally appealing. The leaves of this pretty Malaysian bush carry little indication of their potential, since the scent is only developed through oxidation. The leaves must be fermented and aged before being distilled. Even then, the translucent yellow oil smells harsh. As it ages, it develops patchouli's distinctive scent. Patchouli also has a reputation as an aphrodisiac, a notion that probably originated in India, where it is used as an anointing oil in Tantric sexual practices. All attempts to make a synthetic patchouli have failed.

THERAPEUTIC PROPERTIES

Antidepressant, anti-inflammatory, antiseptic, antiviral, antifungal; reduces fluid retention.

USED FOR

Cosmetically, the essential oil is a cell rejuvenator and antiseptic that treats a number of skin problems, including eczema and inflamed, cracked, and mature skin. As an antifungal, it counters athlete's foot. The aroma helps to relieve headaches, unless the patient doesn't like it!

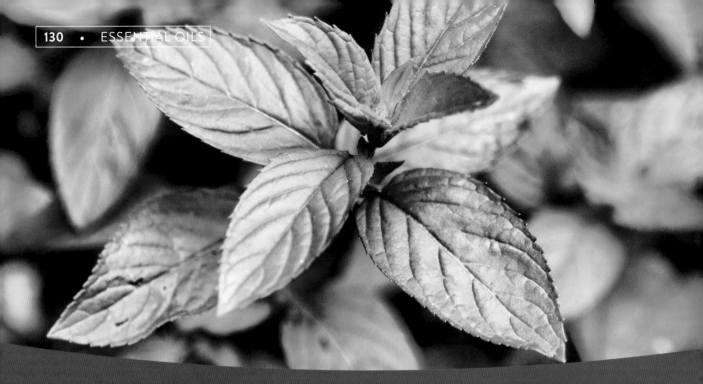

PEPPERMINT

BOTANICAL NAME: *MENTHA PIPERITA*

The most widely used of all aromatic oils, peppermint makes a grand and obvious appearance in all sorts of edible and nonedible products, including beverages, ice cream, sauces and jellies, liqueurs, medicines, dental preparations, cleaners, cosmetics, tobacco, desserts, and gums.

After the *British Medical Journal* noted in 1879 that smelling menthol (the main component in peppermint) relieves headaches and nerve pain, menthol cones that evaporate into the air became all the rage. Taking center stage in several controversies, herbalists have long argued for or against the assertion by the ancient Greek physician Galen that peppermint is an aphrodisiac. But everyone, including modern scientists, agrees that it is a strong mental and physical stimulant that can help one concentrate and stay awake and alert.

THERAPEUTIC PROPERTIES

Anti-inflammatory; relieves pain, muscle spasms, and cramping; relaxes the nerves, kills viral infections, decreases gas and indigestion, clears lung congestion, reduces fever.

USED FOR

Peppermint helps the digestion of heavy foods and relieves flatulence and intestinal cramping, actually relaxing the digestive muscles so they operate more efficiently. A massage over the abdomen with an oil containing peppermint can greatly aid intestinal spasms, indigestion, nausea, and irritable bowel syndrome. Peppermint essential oil is included in most liniments, where it warms by increasing blood flow, relieving muscle spasms and arthritis. Peppermint relieves the itching of ringworm, herpes simplex, scabies, and poison oak. It also clears sinus and lung congestion when inhaled directly. It also destroys many bacteria and viruses. Peppermint is not drying, as one might assume; rather, it stimulates the skin's oil production, so use it blended with other oils to treat dry complexions.

PERU BALSAM

BOTANICAL NAME: *MYROXYLON PEREIRAE*

With a lovely scent of vanilla and spice, Peru balsam is a favorite for use in aromatherapy. The oil comes from a tree in Central and South America, where a legend tells of a wounded Aztec princess who was healed by miraculous balsam resin. The traditional methods of oil extraction are quite interesting: balsam collectors, known as "balsameros," climb the 65-foot-high trunks of the trees and cut the trunks until the resin flows. Cloths are applied to absorb the balsam resin, and they are then combined with bark, pressed, and purified. The purified balsam is then distilled to produce the essential oil.

THERAPEUTIC PROPERTIES

Antioxidant, antiseptic, antibacterial; reduces stress and anxiety; helps eliminate dandruff; useful in dental hygiene.

USED FOR

Helps to eliminate free radicals and prevent infections. The oil has also been shown to repel mites, such as scabies. Peru balsam's calming scent has long been used in aromatherapy to relieve stress and anxiety. A few drops mixed with water and rinsed through the hair can eliminate dead skin cells on the scalp and prevent dandruff. The pleasant scent and taste makes the oil a popular additive to toothpaste and mouthwash.

PRECAUTIONS

Peru balsam is known to be a highly allergenic substance for some people. Always perform a patch test before using the essential oil.

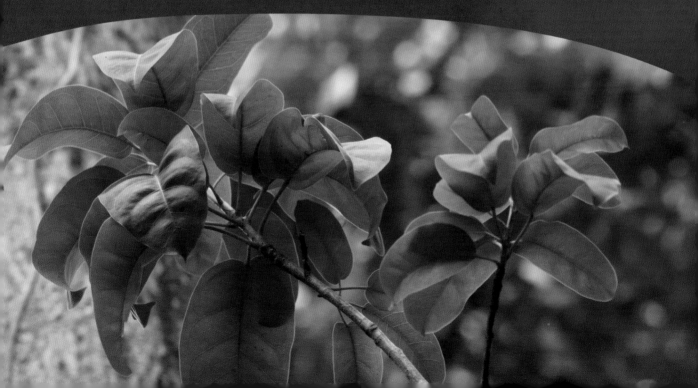

PETITGRAIN

BOTANICAL NAME: *CITRUS AURANTIUM*

Petitgrain essential oil is derived from the bitter orange tree, which is a hybrid between the pomelo and the mandarin. The tree is native to southeast Asia, and was introduced to Spain by the Moors in the 10th century, where it was eventually dubbed Seville orange. Unlike orange essential oil, which is extracted from the fruit's peel through cold compression, petitgrain essential oil is extracted from the leaves, twigs, and green unripe fruit of the bitter orange tree through steam distillation. The vast majority of this oil is used in the food and beverage or perfume and cosmetics industries, but there are some great ways to use petitgrain oil in your own home.

THERAPEUTIC PROPERTIES

Antispasmodic and sedative; good for skin and hair care; eases stress and anxiety, and lowers blood pressure.

USED FOR

Petitgrain is especially known for its soothing, calming properties, and can be used to calm coughs and cramps, as well as promote a good night's sleep. A couple drops of petitgrain can be added to a carrier oil and rubbed on the face to soothe sensitive skin. Or, try adding a couple drops to your shampoo to balance the oil production on your scalp. Used in aromatherapy, petitgrain is excellent for easing stress and anxiety, and helps to lower blood pressure.

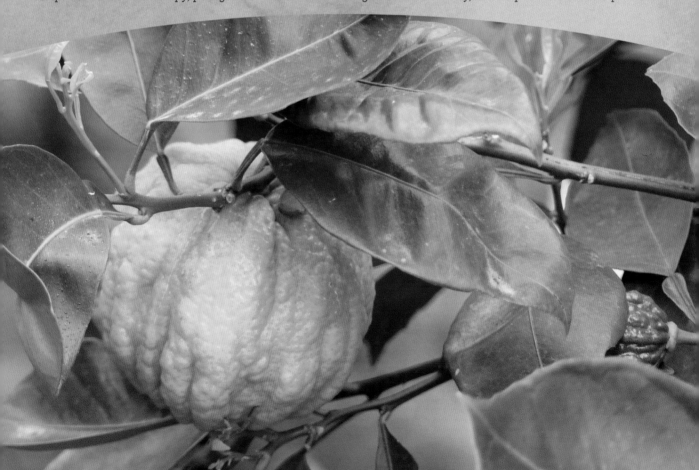

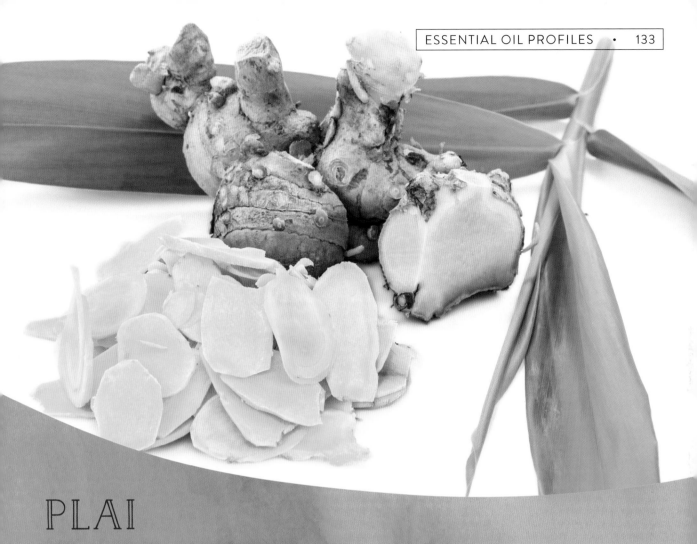

PLAI

BOTANICAL NAME: *ZINGIBER CASSUMUNAR*

Native to Thailand, plai is a species of plant in the same family as ginger. Although it is relatively new to the essential oil scene, it has long been used by Thai massage therapists thanks to its ability to relieve discomfort and inflammation. But unlike ginger's warming effect, plai has a pleasant cooling effect that makes it especially soothing for aches and pains. The oil has a very high concentration of a substance called Terpinen-4-ol, which is the same ingredient that gives tea tree oil its antimicrobial properties—making plai an excellent addition to your healing essential oil arsenal.

THERAPEUTIC PROPERTIES

Anti-inflammatory, antimicrobial; helps ease respiratory problems; antispasmodic.

USED FOR

Plai's anti-inflammatory properties make it especially effective for treating aches and pains associated with muscle pulls and strains. It can be used to prevent infection and treat skin conditions such as acne. When used in a diffuser, plai has been shown to be helpful for asthma, bronchitis, and colds and flu. Its antispasmodic properties help to ease menstrual pain and irritable bowel syndrome.

POPLAR

BOTANICAL NAME: *POPULUS BALSAMIFERA*

There are about 35 different trees in the *Populus* genus that are native to North America, and this large group is loosely divided into cottonwoods, aspens, and balsam poplars. Distilling the sticky, resinous, flowering buds of the balsam poplar is one way to produce the essential oil. While it is one of the rarer and lesser-known oils on the market, the buds of the poplar have been used by Native American medicine men for hundreds of years thanks to the medicinal properties of the buds. In fact, when Europeans first arrived in North America, the native people shared their healing balm with them, which the visitors dubbed "balm of Gilead" after the "healing balm of Gilead" referenced in the Bible.

THERAPEUTIC PROPERTIES

Antiseptic, anti-inflammatory; can help heal scars; analgesic.

USED FOR

The oil helps to heal many skin conditions and injuries, including cuts, bruises, acne, and scars. It has been shown to be an effective remedy for relieving the pain of sore muscles, arthritis, and injuries.

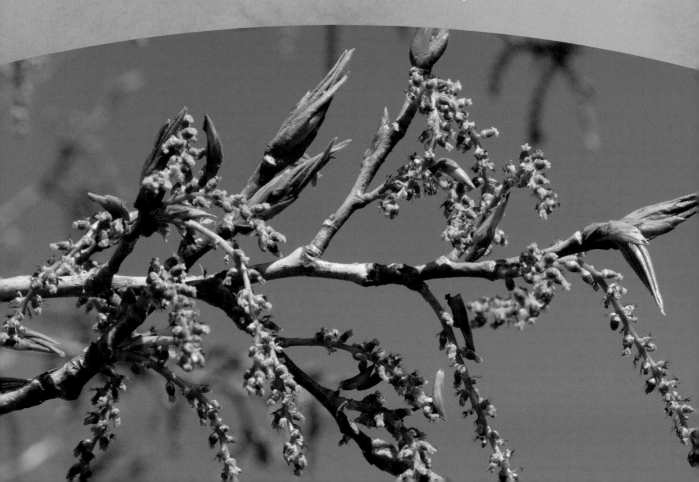

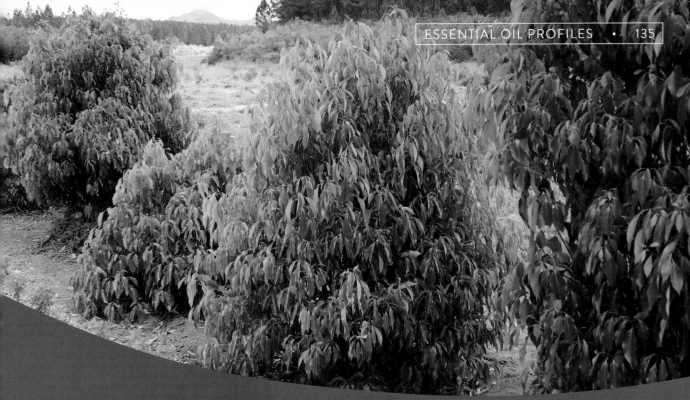

RAVENSARA

BOTANICAL NAME: *RAVENSARA AROMATICA*

Ravensara is distilled from the leaves of a tree that grows in the humid rain forests of Madagascar. The leaves were traditionally burned to help ward off disease. The oil's healing attributes are indeed remarkable, especially when used for respiratory ailments. Aromatherapists recommend having it around during the winter months. Add a few drops to a hot bath or shower, inhale it via diffuser, or simply carry a vial around with you and take a whiff when needed.

THERAPEUTIC PROPERTIES

Antibacterial and antiviral; decongestant; soothes cold sores and shingles; eases digestion.

USED FOR

Ravensara is a must-have for the winter cold and flu season. It enhances immunity-boosting blends and works well with oils like chamomile, cypress, eucalyptus, lavender, lemon, marjoram, niaouli, rosemary, and thyme. It also helps relieve the irritation of chicken pox and shingles.

RAVENSARA OR RAVINTSARA?

It's not just a variant spelling for the same oil—there is an essential oil named ravintsara, and it is a distinctly different oil. Ravintsara is derived from the tree *cinnamomum camphora*. While its therapeutic uses overlap with those of ravensara (via inhalation, it's a great antiviral that can alleviate cold, flu, and respiratory conditions), its chemical profile is different. Correct identification of the two essential oils in the marketplace has been spotty over the past several decades. When you purchase ravensara, make sure that your source identifies the oil as *ravensara aromatica*, and that the retailer clearly distinguishes between the two oils.

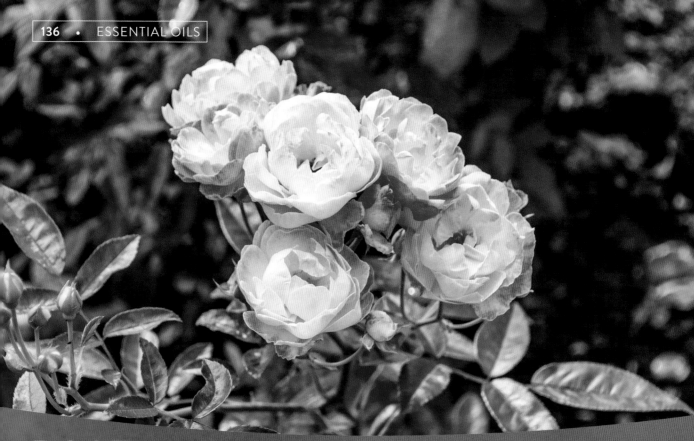

ROSE

BOTANICAL NAME: *ROSA DAMASCENA, R. GALLICA, AND OTHERS*

Originally from Asia Minor, the plant was brought by Turkish merchants to Bulgaria, where the most valued oil is now produced. It is gentle and nontoxic but extremely costly, because so little can be made during distillation and because the bushes need so much care. The oil is distilled or solvent-extracted from blossoms; but, as it is difficult to separate from water, the oil must be distilled at least twice, resulting in two products. The first is called attar of roses; the by-product is called rose water. The unadulterated oil congeals when it cools, but can be liquefied again by the warmth of the hand. It has been an age-old favorite essential oil in facial creams because, in addition to its incredible fragrance, it is reputed to fend off aging. It is also used in costly perfumes.

THERAPEUTIC PROPERTIES

Antidepressant, antiseptic, anti-inflammatory, astringent, antibacterial, antiviral; increases menstruation, calms nervous tension.

USED FOR

A cell rejuvenator and powerful antiseptic, rose essential oil soothes and heals skin conditions, including cuts and burns. It helps a variety of female disorders, possibly by balancing hormones. A massage oil helps various types of female problems, including menstrual cramps, PMS symptoms, and moodiness during menopause. Many women report that simply smelling rose's fragrance is enough to do the trick. Sniffing the oil or using a massage oil containing rose has even been suggested to help reverse impotency.

ROSEMARY

BOTANICAL NAME: *ROSMARINUS OFFICINALIS*

This Mediterranean native with tiny, pale blue flowers that bloom in late winter loves growing by the ocean—its latin name *rosmarinus* means "dew of the sea." It is cultivated worldwide, although France, Spain, and Tunisia are the main producers of the essential oil.

THERAPEUTIC PROPERTIES

Antiseptic, astringent, antioxidant; relieves rheumatic and muscle pain, relaxes nerves, improves digestion and appetite, increases sweating.

USED FOR

As an ingredient in a massage oil, compress, or bath, rosemary essential oil is excellent for increasing poor circulation and easing muscle and rheumatism pain. It is especially penetrating when used in a liniment. It is very antiseptic, so inhaling the essential oil or adding it to a vapor balm that is rubbed on the chest and throat relieves lung congestion and sore throat. It is a stimulant to the nervous system and increases energy. Cosmetically it encourages dry, mature skin to produce more of its own natural oils. It also helps get rid of canker sores. Add it to shampoos—it is an age-old remedy for dandruff and hair loss.

PRECAUTIONS

It can be overly stimulating and may increase blood pressure.

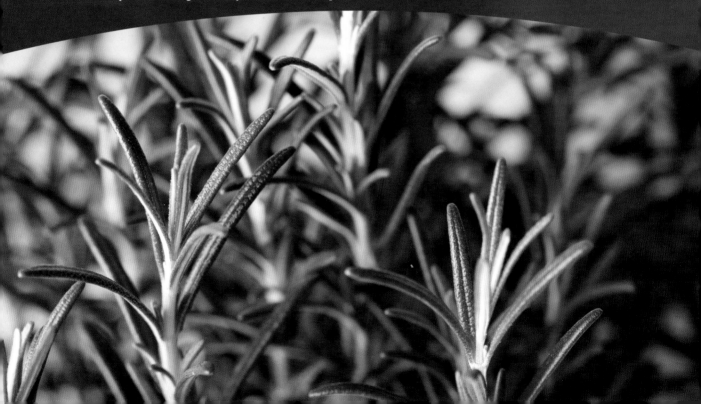

ROSEWOOD

BOTANICAL NAME: *ANIBA ROSAEODORA*

Brazil is famous for its rosewood trees, which can grow to more than 130 feet tall and produce heavy, strong wood that is prized for use in building materials, furniture, and musical instruments. The wood also has a high oil concentration, which produces an essential oil with a lovely rose scent, making it a favorite for perfumes and bath products. But the oil has many health benefits that go beyond its uplifting scent. Be sure to research sources before buying: responsible and reputable rosewood oil distilleries plant new trees for any that are cut down. This is an important step to maintain the beautiful and useful rosewood, which is known as "the ivory of the forest" due to illegal harvesting.

THERAPEUTIC PROPERTIES

Antiseptic; insect repellent; excellent for use in aromatherapy.

USED FOR

Rosewood oil helps cuts and scrapes heal faster and prevents infection. Although less potent than some oils, it can help to relieve headaches, toothaches, and muscle pain. Rubbed on the skin, rosewood can repel mosquitoes. The oil can also be used to kill small insects like bed bugs, fleas, and ants. Its sweet, floral scent makes it a great choice for adding to bath water or a diffuser.

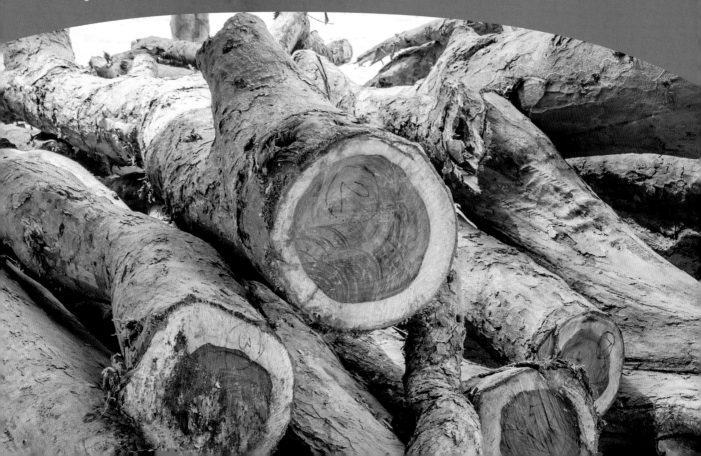

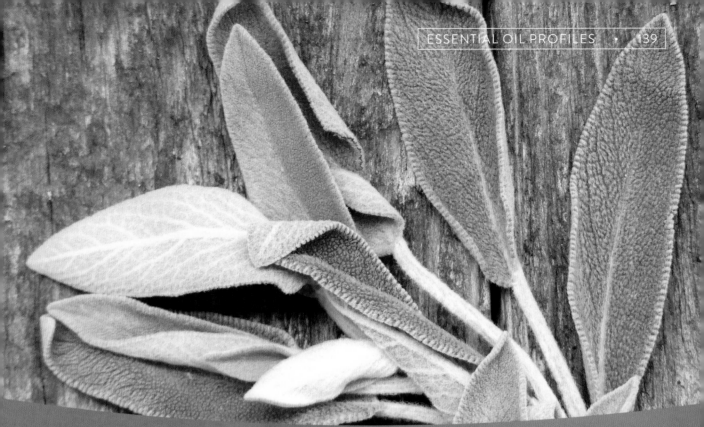

SAGE

BOTANICAL NAME: *SALVIA OFFICINALIS*

Native to the Mediterranean, sage has been known for its medicinal properties since ancient times, when the Greeks and Romans used it as a cure-all for everything from recovering memory loss to preventing plague. In fact, its very name is derived from the Latin *salvere*, which means "to feel healthy" or "heal." This herb is one of the oldest-known plants used not only in medicine, but also in food, and may conjure up memories of holiday tables laden with turkeys and sage stuffing. But the many uses of this ancient oil may persuade you to keep it on hand all year round!

THERAPEUTIC PROPERTIES

Antibacterial, antifungal, antioxidant, anti-inflammatory; helps relieve colds and coughs; eases digestion.

USED FOR

Sage is excellent at preventing infections, both internal and external. Its antioxidant and anti-inflammatory properties make it a valuable ingredient for skin care, as it provides an anti-aging effect and helps fade scars and marks. Sage oil provides relief from coughing and congestion due to colds or flu, and it promotes the production of bile, which helps the digestive system to run smoothly.

PRECAUTIONS

Sage oil is a stimulant, so should be avoided by those with epilepsy. The oil contains camphor, which is toxic in large amounts; always dilute before using, and avoid the oil during pregnancy.

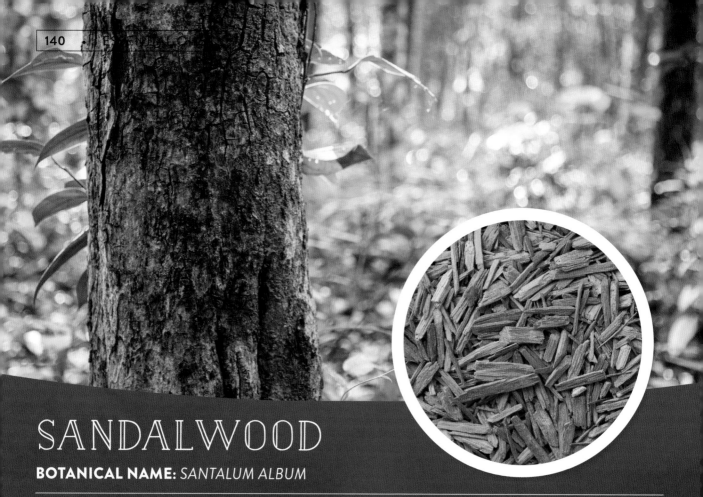

SANDALWOOD

BOTANICAL NAME: *SANTALUM ALBUM*

Sandalwood is distilled from the roots and heartwood of trees that take 50 to 80 years to reach full maturity. In an amazing and lengthy manufacturing process used since ancient times, the mature sandalwood trees are cut down, then left to be eaten by ants, which consume all but the fragrant heartwood and roots. The scent, called *chandana*, is used to induce a calm and meditative state. The lasting fragrance only improves with age. Temple gates and religious statues are carved from the wood because of the exquisite scent and because it is impermeable to termites and other insects. Mysore, India, produces the finest quality oil, and as an endangered species, sandalwood is regulated by the Indian government, which now grows the trees in cultivated plantations.

THERAPEUTIC PROPERTIES

Antidepressant, anti-inflammatory, antifungal, astringent, sedative, insecticide; relieves lung congestion and nausea.

USED FOR

The essential oil treats infections of the reproductive organs, especially in men, and helps relieve bladder infections. For either use, add 12 drops of essential oil for every ounce of carrier oil and use as a massage oil over the infected area. This oil also counters inflammation, so it can be used on hemorrhoids. A syrup or chest balm containing sandalwood helps relieve persistent coughs and sore throat. One of sandalwood's most important uses is to sedate the nervous system, subduing nervousness, anxiety, insomnia, and to some degree, reducing nerve pain. Researchers have found it relaxes brain waves. Suitable for all complexion types, it is especially useful on rashes, inflammation, acne, and dry, dehydrated, or chapped skin.

SCOTCH PINE

BOTANICAL NAME: *PINUS SYLVESTRIS*

You may already be familiar with the Scotch pine tree: it's one of the most common trees used for Christmas trees in the United States. The tree is native to Europe and Asia; in fact, it's the only pine tree native to northern Europe. The beneficial oil derived from the tree has been used since the time of Hippocrates, who took note of its healing effects on the respiratory system. And Native Americans would use mattresses stuffed with pine needles to repel fleas and lice. They were obviously on to something: the highest concentration of Scotch pine's essential oil is found in the fragrant needles.

THERAPEUTIC PROPERTIES

Antibacterial, anti-inflammatory, analgesic, decongestant, deodorizer; useful in aromatherapy.

USED FOR

Scotch pine oil is great for calming skin disorders like acne, eczema, psoriasis, or insect bites. Its anti-inflammatory and analgesic properties can help to reduce pain and swelling from arthritis or injuries. One of its most common uses is in cold and cough remedies: a few drops mixed with coconut oil and rubbed into the chest and neck can help open blocked nasal passages. Its familiar, uplifting scent and antibacterial properties make it a great choice to use as a household cleaner.

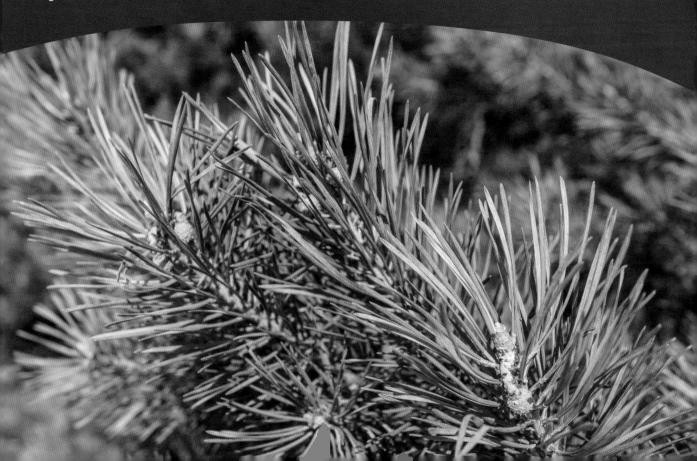

SPEARMINT

BOTANICAL NAME: *MENTHA SPICATA*

What do Moroccan tea, chewing gum, and mojitos all have in common? Spearmint, of course! The popular herbaceous plant is native to Europe and Asia, but is now grown all over the world. And for good reason: not only is the herb commonly used to flavor food and drinks, but spearmint oil has been used medicinally since antiquity. In ancient Greece, spearmint was added to baths and used as a mouthwash. In Ayurvedic medicine, the oil was prescribed to treat digestive conditions, headaches, and skin problems. Spearmint contains menthol, just like its cousin, peppermint, but in a much smaller concentration. This makes it less irritating to the skin, and a great substitute for those who are sensitive to peppermint.

THERAPEUTIC PROPERTIES

Antibacterial, antiviral, and antifungal; helps relax muscles; relieves congestion; insect repellent.

USED FOR

Spearmint oil can be used to prevent infection in cuts, scrapes, and insect bites, and also treat conditions like athlete's foot and dermatitis. The oil can relax muscles to ease aches and pains or calm coughs. A couple drops of spearmint in a diffuser can help relieve congestion due to colds or flu. The oil can be used as an insect repellent to ward off mosquitoes, flies, ants, and moths.

PRECAUTIONS

Pregnant women should not use spearmint oil, as it can possibly cause miscarriage.

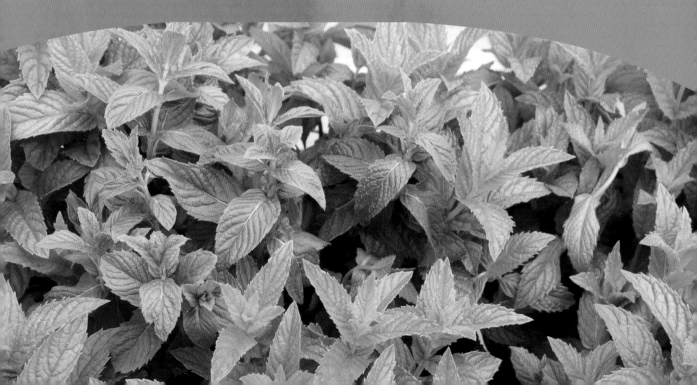

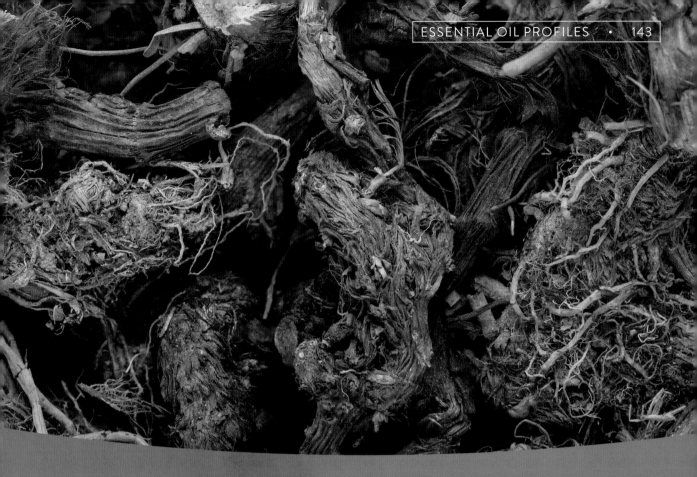

SPIKENARD

BOTANICAL NAME: *NARDOSTACHYS JATAMANSI*

Native to the Himalayas, spikenard is a flowering plant in the honeysuckle family. The roots and stems of the plant have been used since ancient times to create an aromatic oil, which is used for perfumes and medicine. Highly regarded in Indian Ayurvedic medicine, the oil is prized for its effects on depression, anxiety, and insomnia. Spikenard also has religious significance, and is referenced in both the Old and New Testaments of the Bible. Perhaps the most famous biblical reference is in the book of John, when Mary of Bethany spent a year's wages on spikenard ointment to anoint Jesus' feet. Luckily, today we can purchase this beneficial oil without breaking the bank.

THERAPEUTIC PROPERTIES

Antibacterial, anti-inflammatory, antiviral; aids respiratory issues.

USED FOR

Spikenard has been shown to help cuts and scrapes heal faster, and can be used to treat toenail fungus and athlete's foot. Its sedative properties can help those with insomnia fall asleep faster. The oil can be used as a natural laxative to relieve constipation. Spikenard's calming scent relaxes the mind as well as the body, and helps to quell the effects of depression and anxiety.

SPRUCE

BOTANICAL NAME: *PICEA MARIANA* (BLACK SPRUCE)

Thriving in the colder climate of the northern United States and Canada, several species of spruce trees produce essential oils, including the Norway and white spruce varieties. But the species most commonly used for its oil is the black spruce. Traditionally, Native Americans would use spruce mixed with honey to treat skin injuries, as well as using the tree in spiritual ceremonies. Meanwhile, Europeans used spruce to heal gum and stomach infections. Today, the essential oil, which is steam distilled from the needles and twigs of Canadian black spruce trees, is still used for these afflictions, and also has a long history of use in saunas and steam baths.

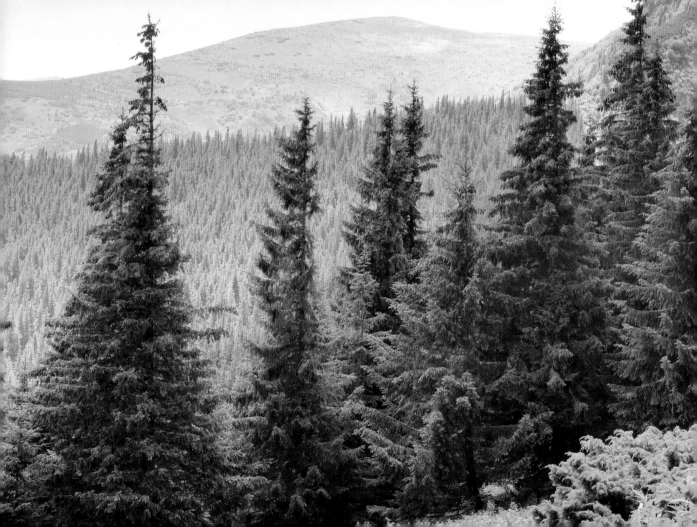

Black spruce essential oil comes from the tree's sharp, bluish-green needles and twigs. It has a refreshing, deep-forest scent, making it useful in aromatherapy for both energizing and calming effects. Via diffuser, it is used for relieving stress and mental fatigue, easing sadness, and providing spiritual uplift. Diluted in a carrier oil, it provides relief for muscle and joint pain, poor circulation, and flexibility issues.

Quite similar to black spruce, Norway spruce (Picea abies) essential oil has a crisp, green, uplifting scent, making it perfect for diffusion, as a cleaning agent for kitchens and bathrooms, as a health restorative, and as an addition to massage oil blends.

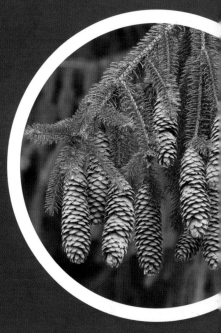

When diffused, the effects of white spruce (Picea glauca) have been described as grounding, centering, healing, uplifting, invigorating, and revitalizing. In fact, its rejuvenating effects on some people can be profound. It is also one of the best spruce oils to assist in breaking up mucus, easing asthma, bronchitis, and coughs, and providing all-around respiratory healing.

In general, the spruce essential oils can be used to speed the healing of minor cuts and scrapes, while preventing infection. A few drops added to a carrier oil and rubbed into muscles or joints can help soothe pain from injuries, strains, and arthritis. Spruce is an excellent oil to add to a steam bath to ease the symptoms of colds and flu. If these essential oils smell very familiar, that's because you've probably smelled them before in household cleaners, soaps, or air fresheners.

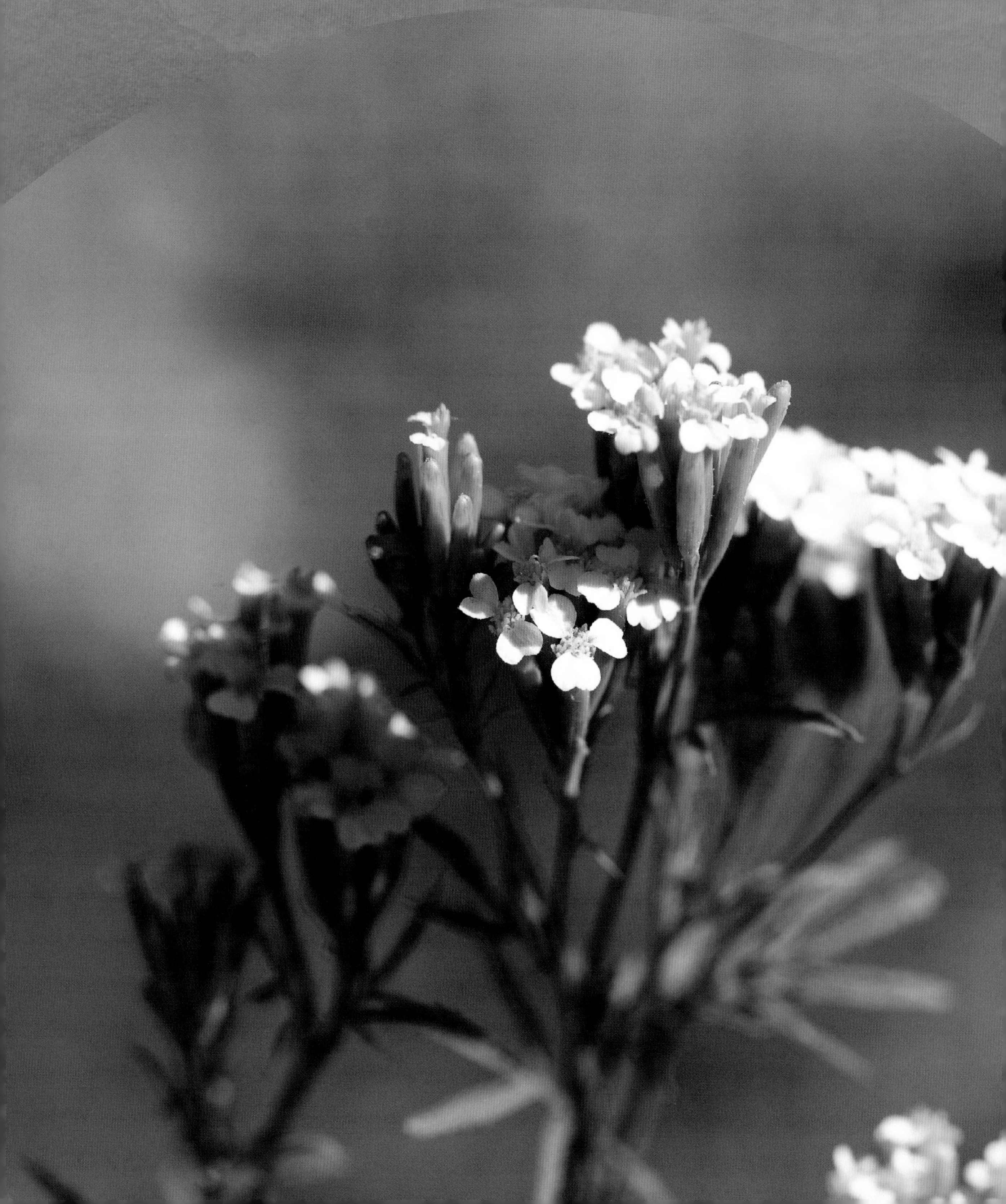

TAGETES

BOTANICAL NAME: *TAGETES MINUTA*

Also known as marigold, tagetes is a plant in the sunflower family native to North and South America; but many species—including *Tagetes minuta*, from which the essential oil is derived—have been naturalized around the world. The flowering plant grows well in just about any kind of soil, and this attribute is what inspired its moniker: *tagetes* is derived from the name of the ancient Etruscan prophet Tages, who was said to have spontaneously sprung out of a plot of plowed ground. Tagetes is used as an herb and flavoring in many South American countries, with a flavor described as a mix between basil, tarragon, mint, and citrus. The essential oil, which is steam distilled from the leaves, stalks, and flowers of the plant, has a sweet, fruity, slightly citrusy scent, and has traditionally been used to treat a myriad of ailments, including colds, whooping cough, colic, and mumps. This oil is often confused with calendula, but don't be fooled: tagetes is a gem in its own right!

THERAPEUTIC PROPERTIES

Antibacterial, antifungal, and anti-inflammatory; sedative; helps relieve respiratory ailments; insect repellent.

USED FOR

Tagetes oil can be used to treat cuts and wounds and prevent infection, and is useful for treating and preventing fungal infections like athlete's foot. Its antibacterial and antifungal properties also make it a great disinfectant for your home, where it can be used to wipe down kitchen and bathroom countertops and floors. With its anti-inflammatory properties, tagetes is a great choice for easing aches and pains in joints and muscles, whether caused by arthritis, rheumatism, or injuries. The oil has sedative effects which can calm coughs and spasms, and also help to relieve anxiety and stress. Tagetes has been used for centuries as a way to ease respiratory ailments, including colds, flu, and bronchitis. Add a few drops of tagetes oil to water and spray around your home to repel insects, including mosquitoes, fleas, and bedbugs. Or simply use in a diffuser to not only keep bugs at bay, but also provide a calming scent.

PRECAUTIONS

Tagetes oil is phototoxic, so avoid direct sunlight for at least 24 hours if used topically.

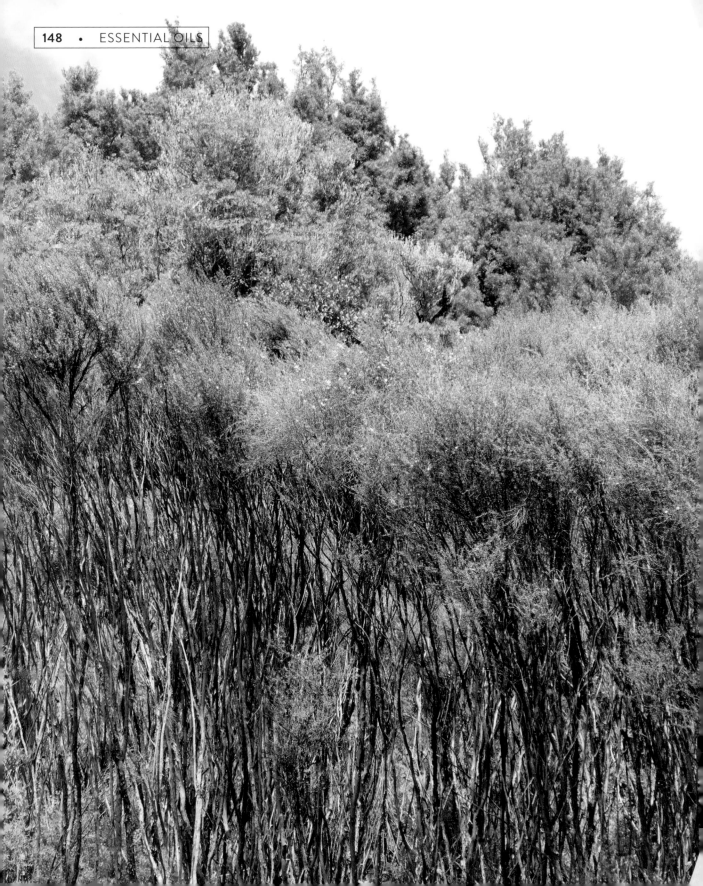

TEA TREE

BOTANICAL NAME: *MELALEUCA ALTERNIFOLIA*

On his first voyage to Australia, Captain Cook made a sharp-tasting tea from tea tree leaves and later used them in brewing beer. Eventually the leaves and then the essential oil were used to purify water. Australian soldiers and sailors used the essential oil as an all-purpose healing agent during World War II.

It's only recently, however, that essential oil companies have begun touting tea tree's healing properties. Medical journal articles support reports of its ability to heal mouth infections, and its primary use is in products for gum infection and canker sores, germicidal soaps, and deodorants. You will find several variations of tea tree, such as the harsher cajuput (*M. cajuputii*) and niaouli (*M. viridiflora*), favored for treating viral infections such as herpes. There is also a tea tree oil that is simply called MQV (*M. quinquenervia viridiflora*). Although it is more expensive, some aromatherapists prefer its softer, sweeter fragrance.

Tea tree essential oil is sometimes sold under its botanical name, Melaleuca.

A MEDICINE CABINET IN A BOTTLE

Tea tree is effective against bacteria, fungi, and viruses and stimulates the immune system. Use it in compresses, salves, massage oil, and washes to fight all sorts of infections, including herpes, shingles, chicken pox, candida, thrush, flu, cold, and those of the urinary tract. Studies show that the presence of blood and pus from infection only increase tea tree's antiseptic powers. It heals wounds, protects skin from radiation burns from cancer therapy, and encourages scar tissue to regenerate. Tea tree also treats diaper rash, acne, wounds, and insect bites. Adding just one drop to dish and diaper washing rinses gets rid of bacteria. It is one of the most nonirritating antiseptic oils, but this varies with the species, so a few people do find it slightly irritating.

MOLD DESTROYER

Add a teaspoon of tea tree oil, 10 drops of clove oil, and a cup of water to a spray bottle and shake thoroughly. Spray the mixture on moldy areas in the bathroom and kitchen. Leave it on for 10 or more minutes and then wipe it away. Tea tree oil can also be used as a mold preventative in toilets, tubs, and shower curtains.

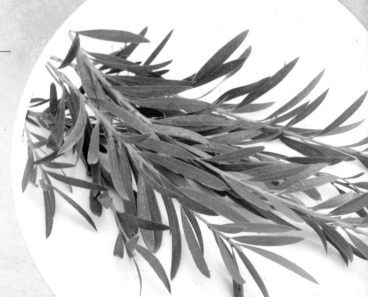

THYME

BOTANICAL NAME: *THYMUS VULGARIS*

Most people consider this low-growing perennial evergreen no more than a culinary seasoning, yet its fragrance led Rudyard Kipling to write of "our close-bit thyme that smells like dawn in paradise."

Thyme was used in Muslim countries for fumigating houses; frankincense was added when people could afford it. The compound thymol, derived from thyme essential oil, is one of the strongest antiseptics known and has been isolated as an ingredient in drugstore gargles, mouthwashes, cough drops, and vapor chest balms. Some of the best-known products that contain thymol are Listerine mouthwash and Vicks VapoRub.

THERAPEUTIC PROPERTIES

Antiseptic, antibacterial, antifungal, antioxidant, astringent; destroys parasitic infections, helps dissipate muscle and rheumatic pain, stops coughing, decreases gas and indigestion, stimulates menstruation, clears lung congestion, stimulates the immune system and circulation.

USED FOR

Thyme essential oil is primarily used in a compress or sometimes in a salve or cream to fight serious infection. It is also useful for treating gum and mouth infections, such as thrush.

PRECAUTIONS

Thyme essential oil can irritate the skin and mucus membranes as well as raise blood pressure, so be sure to use it only in very low dilutions. Red thyme oil is even stronger than the white and is rarely used, except in a liniment for its increased heating effects. Essential oils of thyme are sometimes available in which the most potent components, thymol and carvacrol, are removed, although this decreases their antiseptic properties. Thyme essential oil should not be used with pregnant women or children. Thyme does destroy intestinal worms, but the essential oil should never be taken internally. Instead, use the herb itself in the form of a tea or tincture.

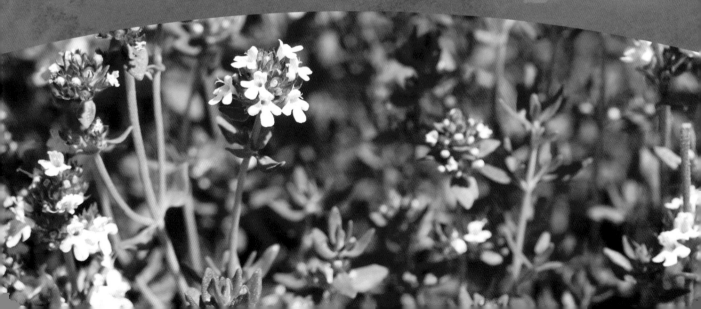

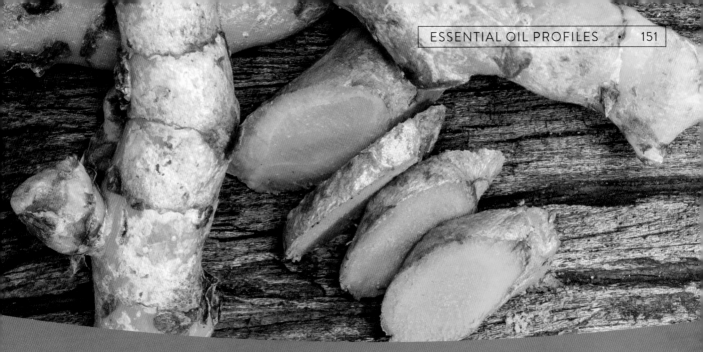

TURMERIC

BOTANICAL NAME: *CURCUMA LONGA*

A member of the ginger family, turmeric is native to Southeast Asia, where it is commonly used in cooking and for dyeing fabrics. But is has also been a staple in traditional medicine for thousands of years. The compound that gives the plant its distinctive yellow color, curcumin, also gives the essential oil powerful healing benefits. But curcumin isn't the only molecule in turmeric with healing properties: the plant is packed with such exotic-sounding substances as sesquiterpenes, borneol, and valeric acid, to name a few. They all work together to give turmeric its much-lauded anti-inflammatory and antioxidant qualities. And as an inexpensive and widely available essential oil, turmeric is a must-have for your medicine cabinet.

THERAPEUTIC PROPERTIES

Antioxidant, anti-inflammatory; helps to lower blood sugar and lowers blood pressure; supports the immune system.

USED FOR

Turmeric is especially prized for its anti-inflammatory properties, making it a great choice for soothing arthritis, muscle pain, headaches, and gastrointestinal inflammation. A few drops in a carrier oil applied to the skin can improve elasticity and reduce wrinkles, thanks to turmeric's antioxidant effects. When ingested in small quantities, turmeric oil helps to ward off infection and support the body's immune defenses. And research shows that turmeric can improve metabolic function in diabetics, as well as boost heart health.

PRECAUTIONS

Ingesting too much turmeric oil can cause stomach upset—use it in moderation. Because of its ability to lower blood pressure, avoid using turmeric if you are on blood pressure medication, as it can cause dangerously low blood pressure.

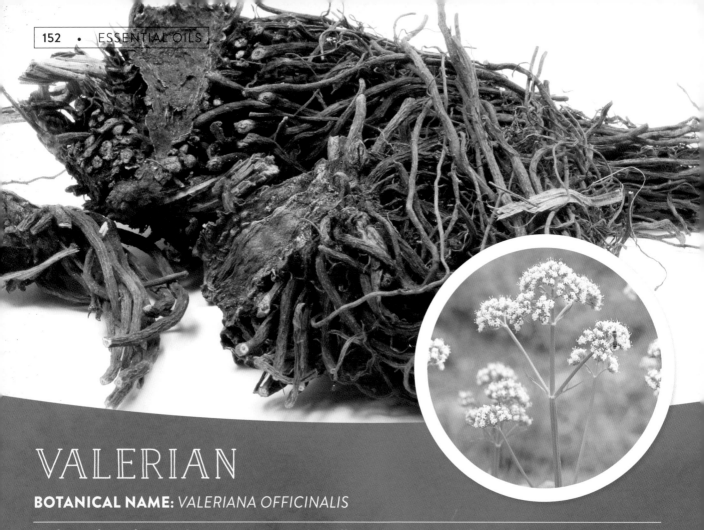

VALERIAN

BOTANICAL NAME: *VALERIANA OFFICINALIS*

Used in perfumes for more than 500 years, sweetish-smelling valerian is a pink-flowered plant native to Europe and parts of Asia. Its scent is appealing to some, but be aware that the musky aroma doesn't appeal to everyone. In fact, the smell can be reminiscent of unwashed socks!

Valerian has been used medicinally at least since the time of the ancient Greeks, and this is where it really shines. The herb was prescribed for insomnia, migraines, and general aches and pains, and the leaves and roots were often boiled and sipped as herbal tea. Even Hippocrates, the "Father of Medicine," lauded its uses. Today, valerian is often used for its relaxing properties, but try it for skin care and digestive health, too!

THERAPEUTIC PROPERTIES

Sedative; reduces stress and anxiety; eases indigestion; good for skin care.

USED FOR

Valerian is probably best known for its calming effects. A couple drops used in a diffuser before bed can help promote and restful night's sleep. This same property can also help relieve stress and anxiety, and possibly lower blood pressure. The oil helps to calm the digestive tract and relive upset stomach, diarrhea, and constipation. Valerian is great for skin health: add a couple drops to a carrier oil and rub over skin to prevent wrinkles and calm conditions like eczema and acne.

VETIVER

BOTANICAL NAME: *CHRYSOPOGON ZIZANIODES*

Native to India, vetiver is a fragrant grass often grown as a barrier to protect crops from pests and weeds. Its lovely, musky, lemony scent has made it a favorite in the perfume industry. In fact, the scent of vetiver is included in 90 percent of perfumes and colognes sold in the West! But this grass is more than just a bug barrier and a pretty scent: vetiver has been used in traditional medicine in Asia and Africa for thousands of years. The essential oil is famous for its soothing, healing properties, and is known as "the oil of tranquility" in India and Sri Lanka.

THERAPEUTIC PROPERTIES

Antibacterial, anti-inflammatory; sedative; helps heal and fade scars.

USED FOR

Vetiver has been shown to stop the growth of bacteria and prevent infection, both when used topically and when ingested. The oil has a soothing and cooling effect, providing relief from aches and pains, and preventing overheating. Its sedative properties can help treat insomnia or anxiety. Vetiver has the ability to regenerate skin tissue, so try adding a few drops into a carrier oil or your favorite lotion and rubbing into scars and marks to help them fade.

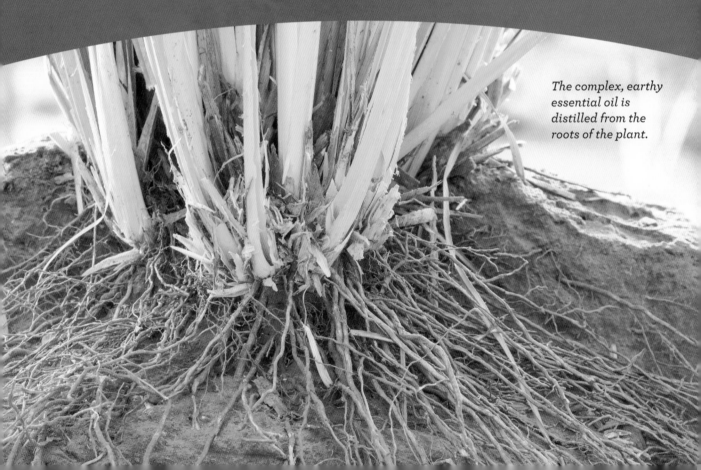

The complex, earthy essential oil is distilled from the roots of the plant.

WINTER SAVORY

BOTANICAL NAME: *SATUREJA MONTANA*

Although closely related to summer savory, winter savory is considered more beneficial for its essential oil. But ironically, winter savory is harvested in the summer, when its pale pink or white flowers are in bloom. The ancient Greeks and Romans used the herb to flavor meat, and considered it an aphrodisiac. Throughout the Middle Ages, winter savory gained popularity in Europe, where it was considered a treatment for gout, mouth ulcers, and toothaches. In fact, the French loved the herb so much that they created a special feast in honor of winter savory, which is still celebrated in Montpellier every December 28.

THERAPEUTIC PROPERTIES

Antibacterial, antifungal, and antiviral; eases digestion.

USED FOR

Winter savory has a high phenol content, which gives it many antiseptic properties. This makes it useful for treating cuts, scrapes, and bug bites. It can also help calm upset stomach, and ease gas, constipation, or diarrhea.

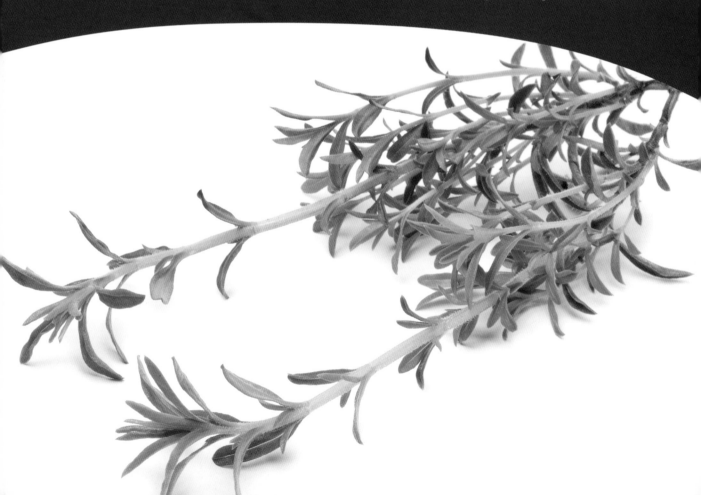

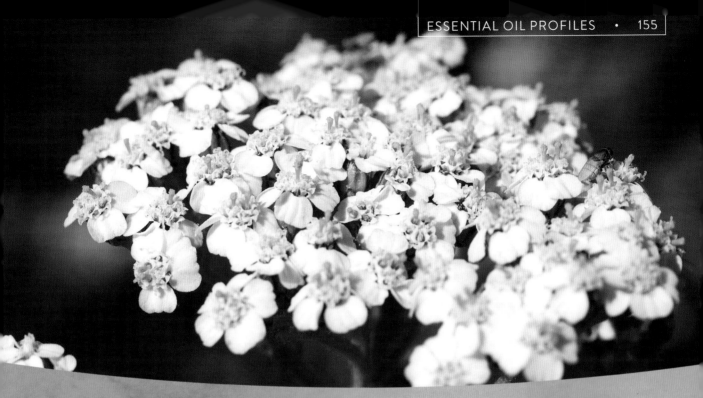

YARROW

BOTANICAL NAME: *ACHILLEA MILLEFOLIUM*

Yarrow, a flowering plant native to Europe, Asia, and North America, has been prized since antiquity for its ability to stanch the flow of blood from wounds. Its botanical name, *Achillea millefolium*, comes from the Greek warrior Achilles, who was said to have used yarrow to treat soldiers on the battlefield. This healing effect of yarrow has resulted in many colorful nicknames for the plant, including soldier's woundwort, nosebleed, bloodwort, and stanchweed. It has also been used in traditional medicine to relieve pain, reduce fever, and treat burns. Today, yarrow essential oil—which is a lovely blue color thanks to the presence of the compound chamazulene—is used for everything from treating wounds to easing digestion.

THERAPEUTIC PROPERTIES

Astringent; antibacterial, antifungal, antiviral, and anti-inflammatory.

USED FOR

Yarrow's claim to fame is its astringent property, which not only helps to stop wounds from bleeding, but also tightens up skin, and may even help prevent hair loss. Yarrow kills microbes of many kinds, preventing infections in cuts and scrapes. Its anti-inflammatory properties help calm aches and pains, and ease swelling of nasal passages due to colds or flu.

PRECAUTIONS

Prolonged exposure to yarrow in high concentrations can induce headaches. Always dilute and use sparingly.

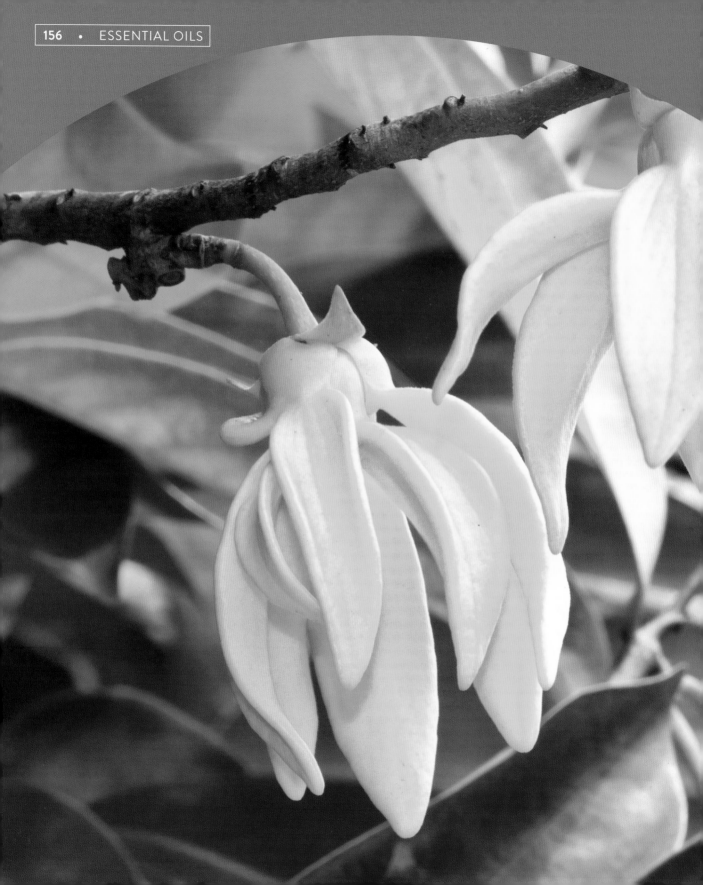

YLANG YLANG

BOTANICAL NAME: *CANANGA ODORATA*

This fragrance is traditionally used to sharpen the senses and to temper depression, fear, anger, and jealousy. For these reasons, and also because of its reputation as an aphrodisiac, the flowers are spread on the beds of the newly married in Indonesia. Modern aromatherapists find the scent strongly sedating, easily sending the most reluctant sleeper off to dreamland. Science, on the other hand, regards ylang ylang more as a mental stimulant. Can it be both? Quite possibly it stimulates people's minds in one way while relaxing them in another.

THERAPEUTIC PROPERTIES

Antidepressant; stimulates circulation, relieves muscle spasms, lowers blood pressure, relaxes nerves.

USED FOR

Of all the essential oils, ylang ylang is one of the best at relaxing the mind and the body. Simply sniffing it can slightly lower blood pressure, although taking a bath with the oil or using it in a massage oil greatly enhances the relaxation experience. It can be helpful in cases of stress, shock, or anxiety. When used as a hair tonic, it balances oil production. Add about 6 drops to every ounce of hair conditioner.

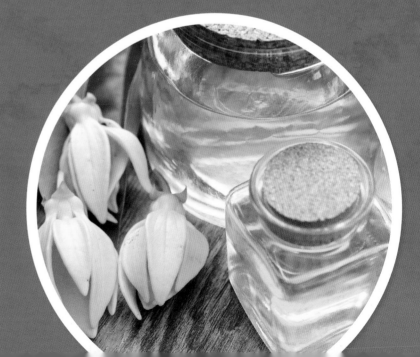

THE ART OF BLENDING

Essential oils vary in odor intensity, which may or may not correspond to the evaporation rate of the aroma notes. Add much smaller amounts of strong essential oils, as it is extremely easy for an especially potent oil such as rosemary to completely overpower the soft scent of an oil such as sandalwood or cedar. When mixing small experimental quantities, one drop of a high intensity oil such as cinnamon can be way too much. Try adding just a smidgen of oil with the end of a toothpick. You can tell which oils have a high odor intensity, such as patchouli and cinnamon, just by smelling them. Use only about one drop of any of these oils to five drops of a more subtle essential oil, such as lavender. On the other hand, orange has such a low odor intensity, you will need about eight drops of it to blend evenly with four drops of lavender.

Here you have the makings of a simple formula: 8 drops orange, 4 drops lavender, and 1 drop clary sage. This combination presents a lesson in intensity and is arranged by notes. The scent leans toward the top and middle note regions. The orange brings sunny brightness to the top, evaporating relatively quickly, while the clary sage provides a sweetly sauntering base for comforting lavender.

There are many ways to alter the formula. For instance, add a drop of cinnamon instead of the clary sage for a scent that's a little more spicy and stimulating. If you want the woodsy smell of cedar, add several drops to balance the blend. The options are almost endless.

Another way to expand a blend is to choose oils that have similar characteristics. It will make your blend seem more complicated and mysterious because no one can pinpoint exactly what the aroma is. Try combining peppermint and spearmint, lemon and bergamot, or cinnamon and ginger. Using oils that come from different parts of a plant tends to deepen and enrich the scent. For instance, add just the tiniest amount of turpentine-like juniper needles to a rich juniper berry to create a more detailed fullness.

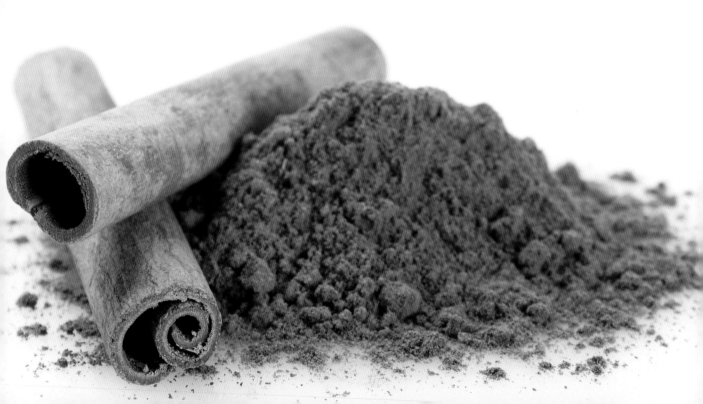

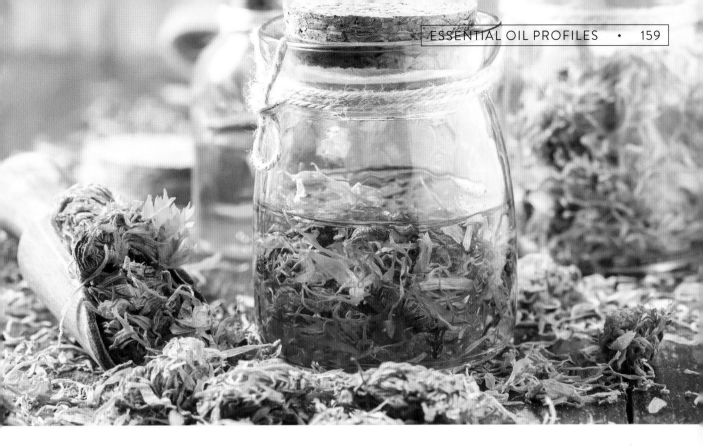

INCORPORATING HERBS

Herbs can be important and effective adjuncts to aromatherapy treatments. In fact, herbs and essential oils used together provide greater healing benefits than does either one alone. The herbs will lend their own less concentrated but more complete medicinal properties.

Oils made by macerating (soaking) herbs in carrier oils are called infused oils. These can replace plain carrier oils in aromatherapy preparations to make a more potent medicine. You can buy an infused oil or make your own.

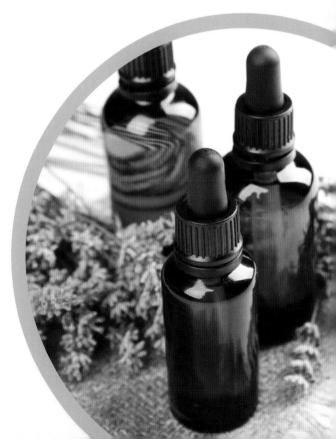

Buying an herbal salve, lotion, or cream and stirring essential oils into it is a quick way to make an herb and essential oil combination. Try to find herbal preparations that contain little or no essential oil, because you don't want to end up with too much essential oil in your final product.

DIFFUSION

Diffusers are small electrical units that release water-based essential oil vapor into a room. Because they are unheated, the volatile compounds in the oils remain intact. Nebulizers also pump essential oil vapor into the air, but do it without water. Generally, you place a few drops of essential oil in a hand-blown glass container and turn on a small compressor that's connected with a piece of tubing. The glass unit disperses a fine mist of micro-particles mixed with the stream of air produced by the pump. This method increases the surface area of the scent molecules. It's an extremely effective way to disinfect and energize the atmosphere. Diffusers and nebulizers can be used in a sick room for 10 to 15 minutes every hour to clear airborne microbes that may spread infection.

Ceramic or metal rings designed to be placed directly on light bulbs are available online and at many stores. Place 2–3 drops on the ring while it's cold, and be sure not to touch it again until it cools down after turning off the light. You can also place a couple drops of essential oil directly on the bulb, although the oil doesn't last as long.

Clay and terra cotta discs and holders are the simplest of all. Add a few drops of oil to the disc surface and allow natural sunlight to heat up the surface and disperse the scent.

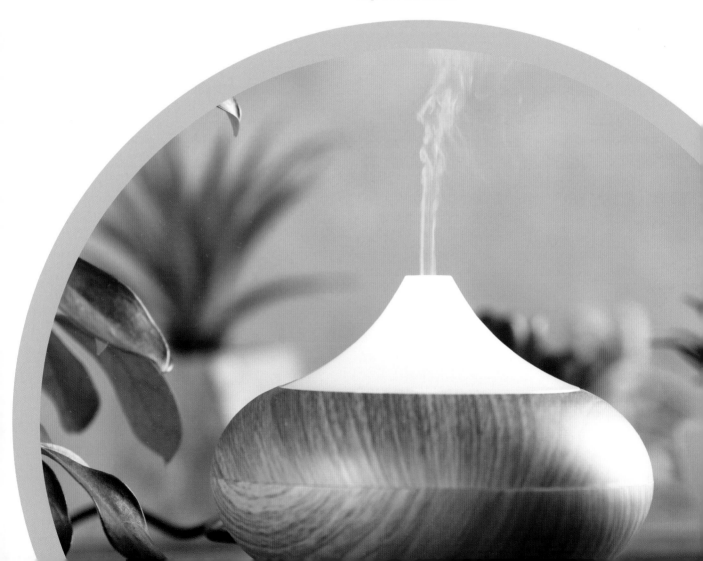

SLEEP TIGHT

- 3 drops chamomile oil
- 3 drops lavender oil
- 3 drops orange oil

Combine all essential oils and add to a diffuser.

The scents of lavender, orange, and chamomile have proven to be effective at reducing stress and anxiety. Use this calming blend before bedtime to help you relax and fall asleep.

FRESH AND CLEAN BLEND

- Bergamot oil
- Grapefruit oil
- Lemon oil
- Lime oil
- Orange oil

Combine one to two drops of each essential oil and add to a diffuser.

With so many bright, cheerful aromas, this blend will make your house smell like you've freshly cleaned! And the lively citrusy scents help to purify the air and uplift your mood.

BREATHE EASY

- 2 drops eucalyptus oil
- 2 drops lemon oil
- 2 drops peppermint oil
- 1 drop clove oil
- 1 drop lime oil
- 1 drop rosemary oil

Combine all essential oils and add to a diffuser.

This blend is perfect to use during cold and flu season. The oils work together to protect against infection, support respiratory function, and clear up congestion.

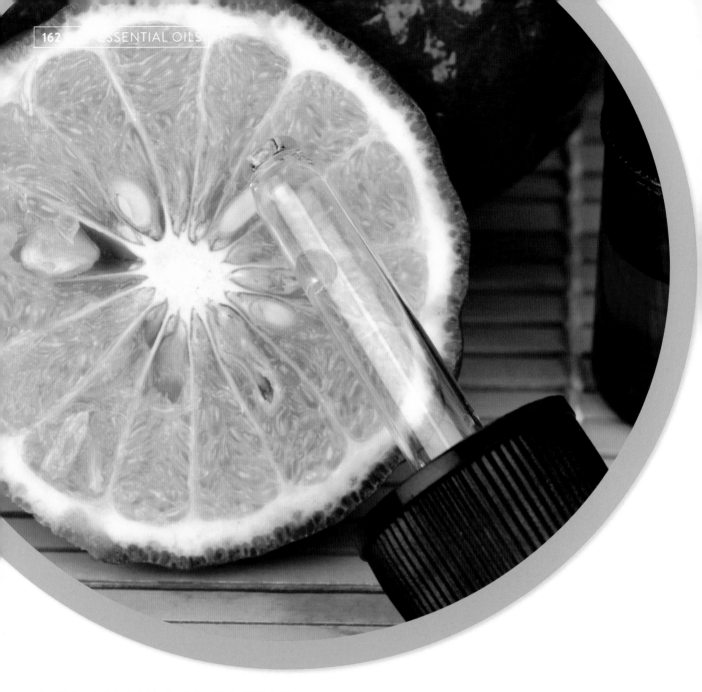

RELAXATION BLEND

- 4 drops lavender oil
- 3 drops clary sage oil
- 2 drops ylang ylang oil
- 1 drop marjoram oil

Combine all essential oils and add to a diffuser.

Had a stressful day? Mix up this relaxing recipe and breathe deeply. All of the oils in this blend have been shown to quell anxiety, promote calm, and reduce blood pressure.

BETTER THAN ASPIRIN

Combine all essential oils and add to a diffuser.

- 6 drops peppermint oil
- 4 drops eucalyptus oil
- 2 drops myrrh oil

Peppermint is more than just a holiday dessert favorite: the cooling scent has been shown to fight off headaches. Together with anti-inflammatory eucalyptus and myrrh, this oil calms pain and nausea, helping you to feel better naturally and without the use of drugs.

UNWANTED GUEST

- 4 drops peppermint oil
- 4 drops spearmint oil
- 4 drops vetiver oil
- 1 drop lemongrass oil

Combine all essential oils and add to a diffuser.

No one wants insects in their home, but spraying chemicals in the air isn't ideal, either. Instead, try diffusing this blend, which contains four potent insect-repelling essential oils. Bonus: your house will smell great, too!

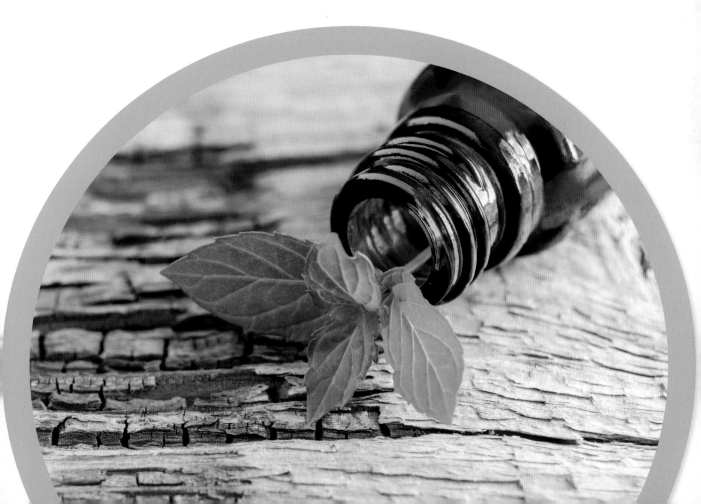

TRANQUIL EVENING

Combine all essential oils and add to a diffuser.

- 3 drops lavender oil
- 3 drops vetiver oil
- 2 drops frankincense oil

This blend combines the relaxing, calming scents of lavender and frankincense with vetiver—known in India as the "oil of tranquility." Try it before bedtime to promote a sense of calm and security.

HAPPY HOLIDAYS

Combine all essential oils and add to a diffuser.

- 3 drops cinnamon oil
- 3 drops orange oil
- 2 drops clove oil
- 1 drop cardamom oil
- 1 drop ginger oil

Instead of burning sooty candles or spraying air fresheners full of chemicals, try a festive blend of essential oils this holiday season. This bright and spicy mix will fill your home with holiday warmth and cheer, without the unwanted toxins.

HAPPINESS BLEND

Combine all essential oils and add to a diffuser.

- 3 drops bergamot oil
- 3 drops lavender oil
- 2 drops geranium oil

Citrusy bergamot, floral geranium, and aromatic lavender combine to produce an uplifting, calming, and mood-boosting scent, perfect for diffusing in your home when entertaining. Both you and your guests will feel happy and relaxed.

COLD REMEDY

Combine all essential oils and add to a diffuser.

- 5 drops rosemary oil
- 4 drops eucalyptus oil
- 4 drops peppermint oil
- 3 drops cypress oil
- 2 drops lemon oil

If you prefer to try natural remedies before perusing the pharmacy's cold medicine aisle, this blend is for you. Rosemary calms aches and pains and relieves nausea, while eucalyptus and peppermint help ease congestion. Cypress helps quell coughs, and a bit of lemon fights fatigue. Everything you need in a cold remedy in one blend!

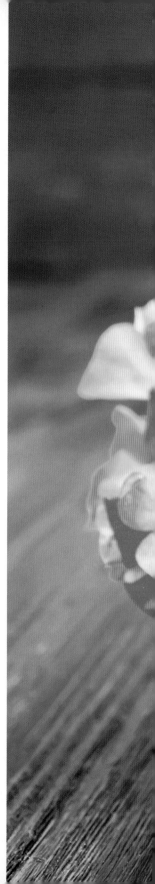

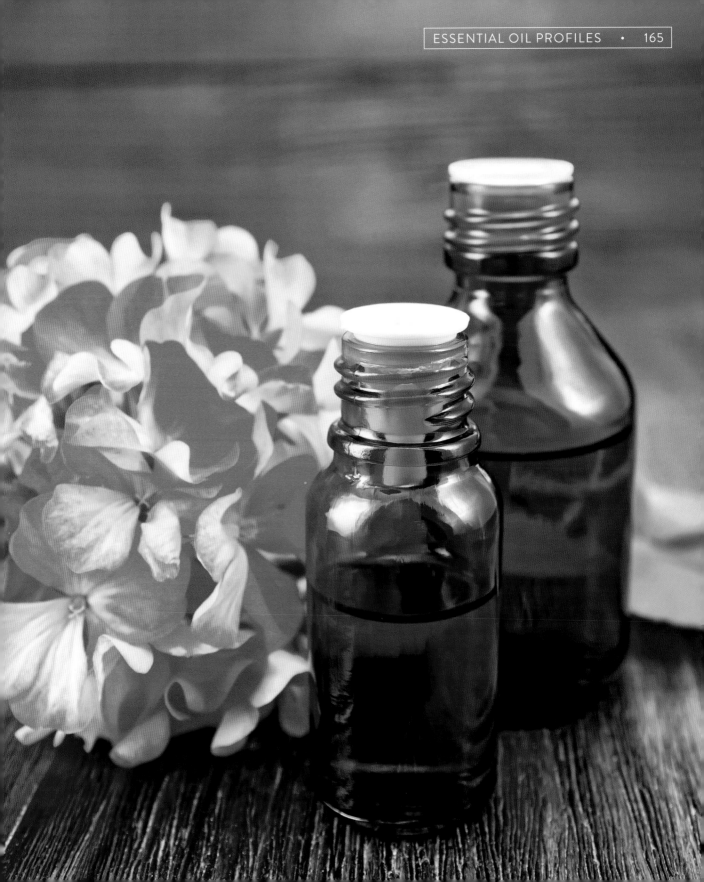

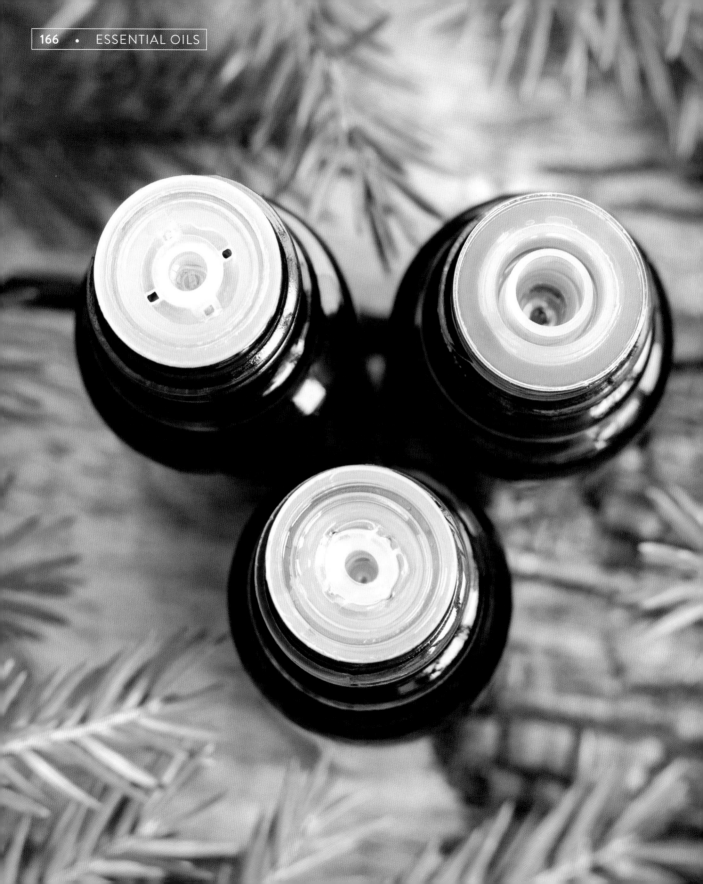

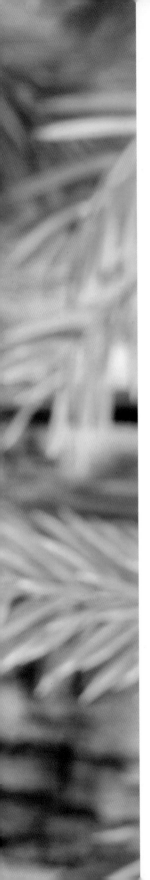

SPRING FLOWERS

- 3 drops chamomile oil
- 3 drops lavender oil
- 2 drops geranium oil

Combine all essential oils and add to a diffuser.

With its herby, floral notes and uplifting scent, this is the perfect blend to use when the weather starts getting warmer. But you don't have to wait: use it whenever you need some springtime in your life!

CHAI TEA

- 3 drops cardamom oil
- 2 drops cassia oil
- 2 drops clove oil
- 1 drop ginger oil

Combine all essential oils and add to a diffuser.

Caution: this blend smells good enough to drink! With the spicy, warm aroma of chai tea, this is a great blend to use in the kitchen. But it doesn't just smell good: the oils in this mix are known for their ability to calm nausea and lower blood pressure.

A WALK IN THE WOODS

- 4 drops frankincense oil
- 3 drops fir oil
- 2 drops cedarwood oil

Combine all essential oils and add to a diffuser.

This warm, woody blend promotes feelings of calm and relaxation. Try it in your home or office after a stressful day: the combination of clean, outdoorsy scents will transport you to the peacefulness of nature.

PAY ATTENTION

- 2 drops grapefruit oil
- 2 drops lavender oil
- 2 drops lemon oil
- 2 drops peppermint oil
- 1 drop basil oil
- 1 drop rosemary oil

Having trouble focusing? The oils in this blend help you stay alert, while also decreasing your stress and anxiety so you can concentrate. A great blend for students to use when preparing for an important exam. Or try it at the office when you need to complete a big project.

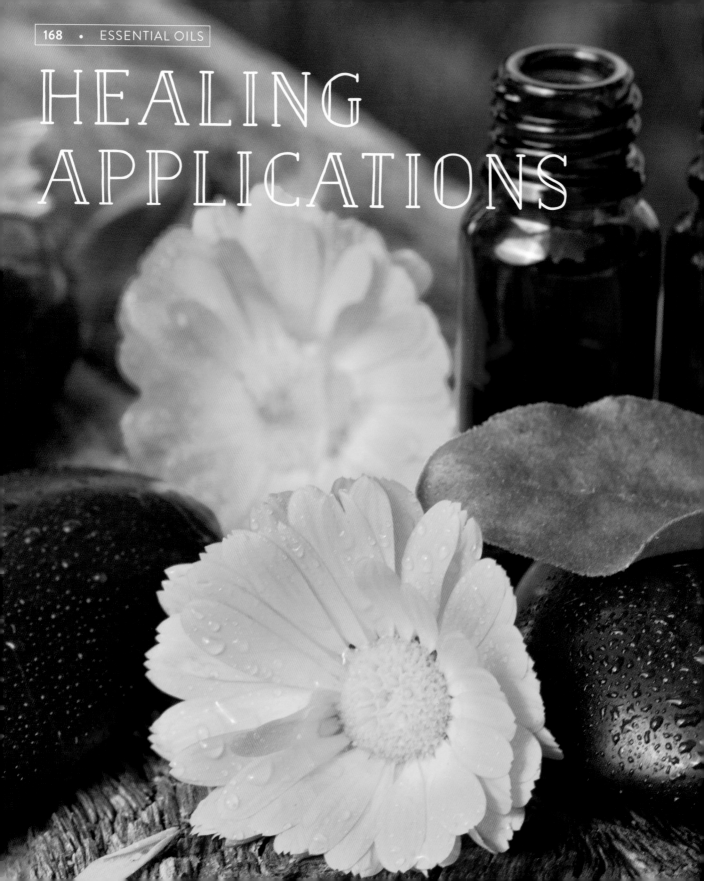

HEALING APPLICATIONS

USING THE REMEDIES

Many remedies given in this chapter are used as a massage or bath oil. That's because the safest way to use essential oils is externally and in a diluted state. You should almost never ingest them. Massage techniques vary—some cover the whole body while others work on only a part of it. Acupressure is an example of a method that requires very little, if any, massage oil. Techniques such as Swedish massage and lymphatic massage call for repeated applications of massage oil. If you find yourself using a tablespoon of massage oil or more at one session, use half the amount of essential oils in the recipe. Remember, the best aromatherapy is achieved when the fragrance is subtle, not overpowering. Cut the amount of essential oils in half when the aromatherapy product will be used on the elderly, children younger than 12 years of age, or someone who is very ill or frail.

Good judgment and common sense are the most important ingredients to use when self-prescribing and treating. Sometimes ailments that seem relatively minor can actually be indications of far more troubling problems. It's a good idea to get professional advice whenever you are in doubt about what you have or how to treat it. Also, don't abandon your prescription drugs in favor of aromatherapy treatments unless you get professional advice that it will be safe to do so.

While aromatherapy offers gentle and effective forms of therapy, you will often get quicker and better results when you combine it with other natural treatments. In many cases, adding herbal remedies, lifestyle changes, and nutritional supplements to your aromatherapy regimen will help you to heal faster and better. In some cases, using the herbs from which the essential oils are made is safer than trying to properly dilute essential oils. This is particularly true when the herb is more effective when it is taken internally. Although you should not ingest essential oils, you can safely drink herb teas such as peppermint to settle your stomach or chamomile to relax you before bed.

Aromatherapy can be a valuable healing tool; however, not all illnesses can be treated with essential oils. Conditions such as diabetes, chronic kidney disease, and multiple sclerosis are not candidates for aromatherapy treatment because they require much more extensive therapy than offered by aromatic chemicals.

HELPFUL HINTS BEFORE YOU BEGIN

- In recipes that call for 12 drops of an essential oil, you might prefer using the equivalent measurement of 1/8 teaspoon.

- If you plan to keep a preparation longer than six months, use one of the longer-lasting, pricier oils (like jojoba). Or add one or two capsules of vitamin E, which will preserve your recipe longer than other oils, but not as long as jojoba.

- When preparing recipes to be used by the elderly, the very young (less than 12 years of age), or anyone who is very ill or frail, be sure to cut the amount of essential oils in half, keeping the carrier (oil, water, alcohol, vinegar, etc.) the same. These people are so sensitive that they will react equally well to the smaller amount.

- Just want to try something out? Make a smaller amount by cutting the proportions in half. If the drops don't divide evenly, use the smaller number. Use a clean toothpick if you only want a smidgen of something, such as patchouli (yes, it's that powerful!).

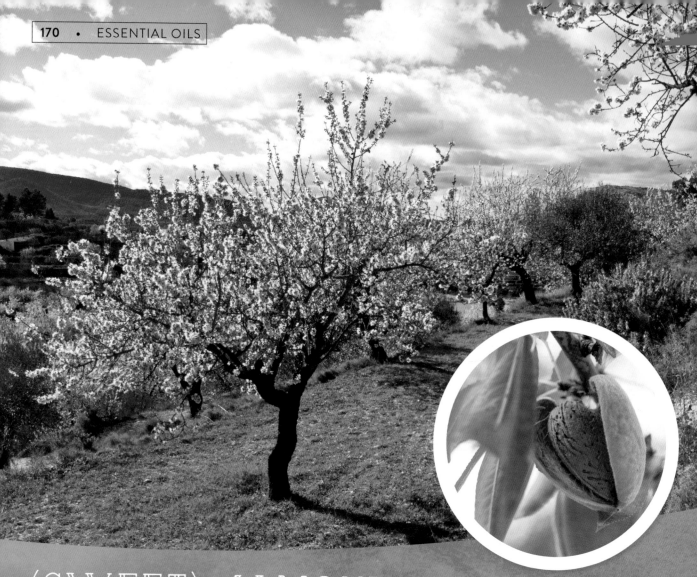

(SWEET) ALMOND OIL

Native to the Middle East and pockets of southwest Asia, almonds have been cultivated and used for oil for centuries. In fact, traditional Chinese, Persian, and Ayurvedic medicine taught about the oil's skin-quenching benefits. Most of the almonds used for oil in the United States come from California, although Marcona almonds, grown in Spain, are also popular. It's not usually necessary to search for "sweet" almond oil, as all of the almonds grown and distributed in the U.S. are sweet almonds. Bitter almonds are known to contain toxic amounts of cyanide, so bitter almond oil should only be used under a doctor's supervision. It should not be used in aromatherapy.

As a carrier oil, sweet almond works well due to its mild scent, which is slightly nutty but not overwhelming. It's also slow to evaporate, and easily absorbed by the skin, giving it great staying power for your essential oils. Even better, the oil is fairly inexpensive and packed with vitamins A, B, and E. One word of caution: sweet almond oil should not be used by those who are allergic to any kind of nuts, as the oil is often produced in the same location as other nut oils.

APRICOT KERNEL OIL

As the name suggests, apricot kernel oil is derived from the kernels—or seeds—of the apricot fruit. The oil has been used for centuries in traditional Chinese medicine, where it is prescribed for tumors and ulcers. Apricot kernel is similar to almond oil in scent and properties, making it another excellent choice for a carrier oil. The oil also possesses many healthy benefits in its own right, giving your essential oils some extra punch.

Some of apricot kernel oil's therapeutic properties include:

Emollient: Apricot kernel oil makes a great moisturizer for your skin.

Anti-inflammatory: The oil reduces inflammation, both internally and externally.

Antibacterial: Like many essential oils, apricot kernel oil also kills harmful bacteria.

Antioxidant and anti-aging: Apricot kernel oil is an excellent choice for skin care, as it helps reduce wrinkles and protects skin against free radicals.

Apricot kernel oil contains oleic and linoleic acids, plus vitamins A and E, making it a popular addition to many expensive skin care products. But you can reap the benefits of this lightweight oil without breaking the bank: most brands can be bought for around $10 a bottle.

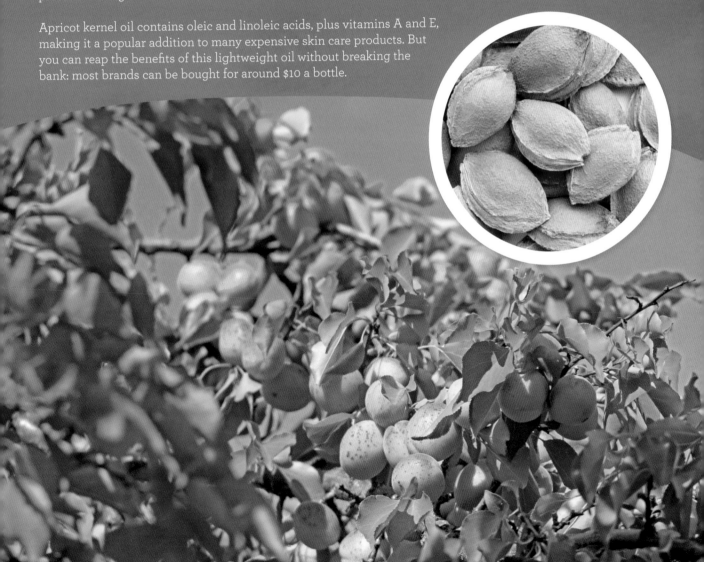

ARGAN OIL

Argan oil is derived from the fruit of the argan tree, a tree that can only be found in Morocco and Algeria. Each fruit contains a nut, which is broken by hand to reveal at least one (and sometimes two or three) oil-rich argan kernels. The kernels are then roasted and ground to express the oil. It can be a long, laborious process; but the oil has become so popular that the Moroccan government plans to increase production of the oil from 2,500 tons to 4,000 tons by the year 2020. And no wonder argan oil is so popular: the oil's high vitamin E content helps to boost cell production in the skin, while moisturizing and easing inflammation. The oil is prized for its ability to increase skin elasticity and soften lines and wrinkles.

Argan oil has a sweet, nutty scent, which can be light or strong, depending on when the oil was harvested. Oil harvested in the spring and summer has a lighter scent, whereas oil harvested in the fall and winter has a more noticeable scent. The oil should be used within six months of opening for the most benefit. Pure argan oil is often more expensive than many oils, due to its scarcity and labor-intensive collection process; but the benefits may be worth it!

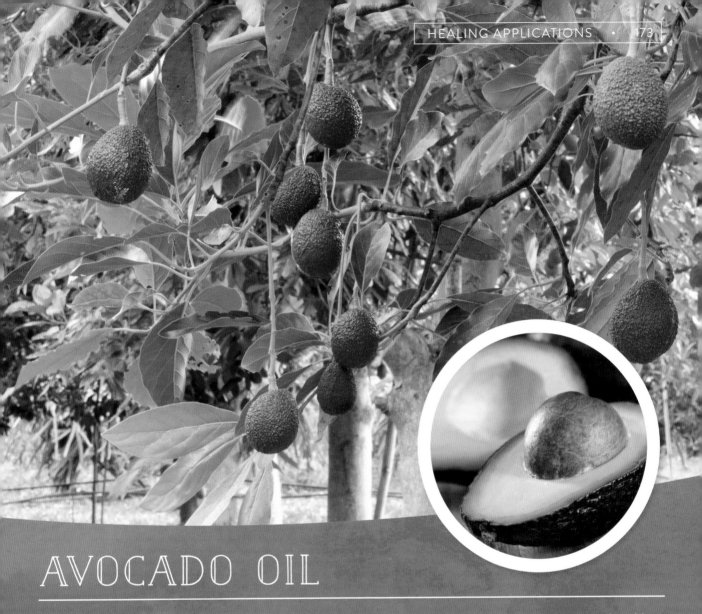

AVOCADO OIL

If you only know the avocado as a guacamole ingredient, you're missing out on an amazing, skin-loving oil! Unlike most other carrier oils, avocado is not extracted from the seed of the fruit, but rather from the fruit itself. After the skins and pits have been removed, avocado flesh is pressed, and then whirled in a centrifuge to separate the pulp from the oil.

The benefits of the emerald green oil have been known since the time of the Aztecs, who used avocado to soften and soothe the skin. Today, we know that the oil is packed with good-for-you ingredients like omega-3 fatty acids, and vitamins A, D, and E. Avocado oil is rapidly absorbed by the skin, but is also thick enough to form a protective barrier. This makes it excellent for treating conditions like psoriasis, and for protecting and healing wounds. It is also considered one of the best oils to use on aging skin, as it contains free-radical-fighting antioxidants and can boost collagen production.

The quality of the oil will depend on the quality of the avocados it is derived from, so search for a reputable brand. For optimal benefits, look for oil that is organic, extra virgin, unrefined, and cold-pressed.

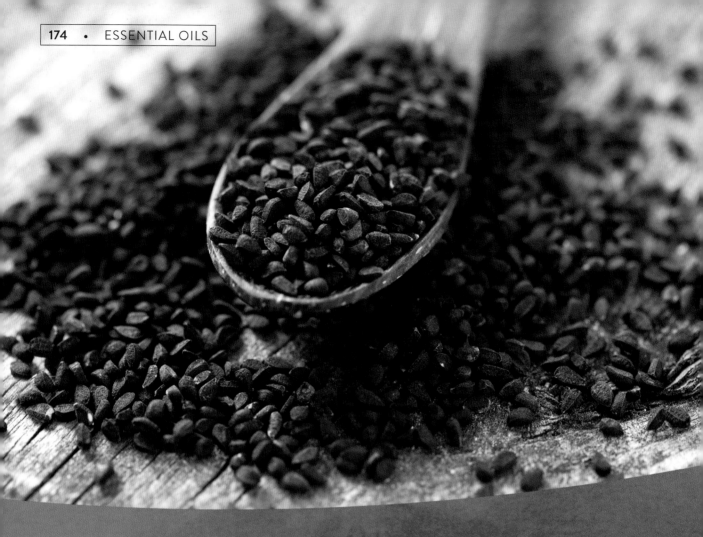

BLACK CUMIN SEED OIL

Black cumin seed oil is often called "the healthiest oil on the planet," yet surprisingly, most Americans have never heard of it. More than 600 scientific articles have been written about the oil, claiming it possesses incredible anti-inflammatory, antibacterial, and antioxidant properties. Studies have shown it to be effective at combating everything from "superbugs" like methicillin-resistant Staphylococcus aureus (MRSA) to autoimmune diseases.

The use of black cumin seed oil dates back to ancient Egypt, and it is said that Cleopatra herself used the oil for her hair and skin. And Hippocrates used black cumin seed to ease digestive troubles. Today, modern science has discovered that the oil contains three beneficial chemicals known as thymoquinone, thymohydroquinone, and thymol. While they may be hard to pronounce—and even harder to spell—these amazing little phytochemicals can work wonders! Not only are they excellent for skin and hair, but they also support the immune system, kill microbes, and ease inflammation.

Black cumin seed oil has a deep, earthy, herbal scent, so it mixes well with essential oils that have strong, woody scents, like juniper berry, sandalwood, and spruce. Be sure to store the oil in a dark glass bottle to protect it from rancidity. This is definitely a carrier oil that should be added to your arsenal!

BORAGE OIL

With one of the highest concentrations of the fatty acid gamma-linolenic acid (GLA), borage oil—also known as starflower oil—is particularly beneficial for dry, mature, sensitive, or damaged skin. The oil is derived from the seeds of the borage plant, which is native to the Mediterranean region. The plant produces lovely blue, pink, and sometimes white flowers, which, like the rest of the plant, are edible. Use of borage as a culinary plant is common in parts of Europe; but the plant is most often grown for its rich oil.

Borage oil has been used since medieval times as a skin moisturizer and a remedy for respiratory issues. The Moorish Arabs brought the herb with them to Spain more than a thousand years ago, making the oil more popular in Europe. It even inspired a poem by Robert Browning with the wordy title, "An Epistle Containing the Strange Medical Experience of Karshish, the Arab Physician." In it, Browning talks about "Blue-flowering borage, the Aleppo sort."

The GLA in borage oil—which makes up about 23 percent of its content—is an omega-6 essential fatty acid which has been found to possess natural anti-inflammatory properties. This makes borage oil another excellent choice for use as a carrier oil.

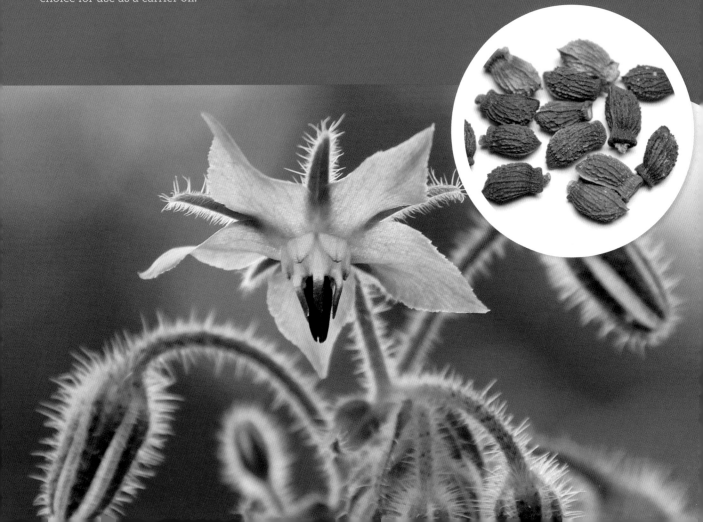

(FRACTIONATED) COCONUT OIL

For thousands of years, indigenous peoples have used the amazing coconut for a myriad of reasons in their daily lives. And coconut oil has enjoyed a surge in popularity in recent years in Western countries. So it should be no surprise that this rich, skin-loving oil is a great choice to use as a carrier oil.

When choosing a carrier oil, we should look for something that mixes well with other oils and quickly and easily penetrates the skin. Extra virgin coconut oil, or unrefined oil, is a solid at room temperature and can't be easily mixed. Instead, look for "fractionated" coconut oil. This oil—sometimes called "liquid coconut oil"—is oil that has been distilled to remove its long-chain fatty acids. This change allows the oil to remain a liquid at room temperature. But not to worry: fractionated coconut oil still contains plenty of medium-chain fatty acids, plus vitamins A, C, and E, all of which help to moisturize the skin and give it a tighter, firmer look.

Coconut oil also has the advantage of having a long shelf life. The oil should last well over five years, so you can enjoy the benefits of this useful oil without worrying about spoilage.

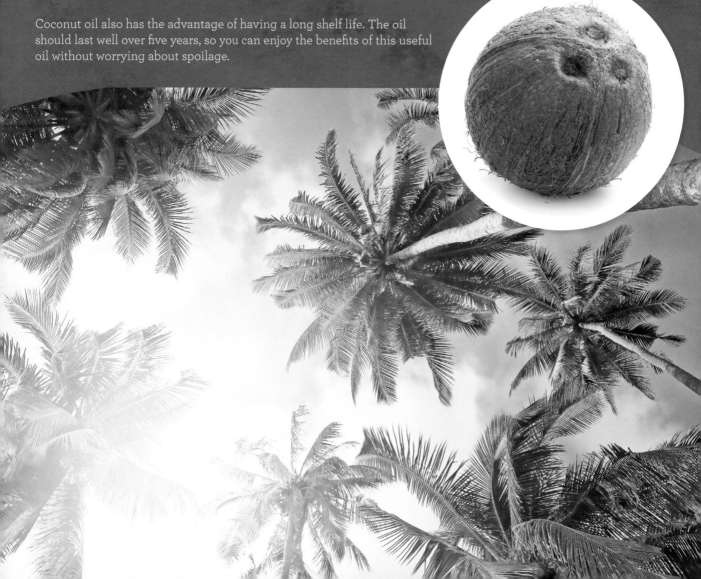

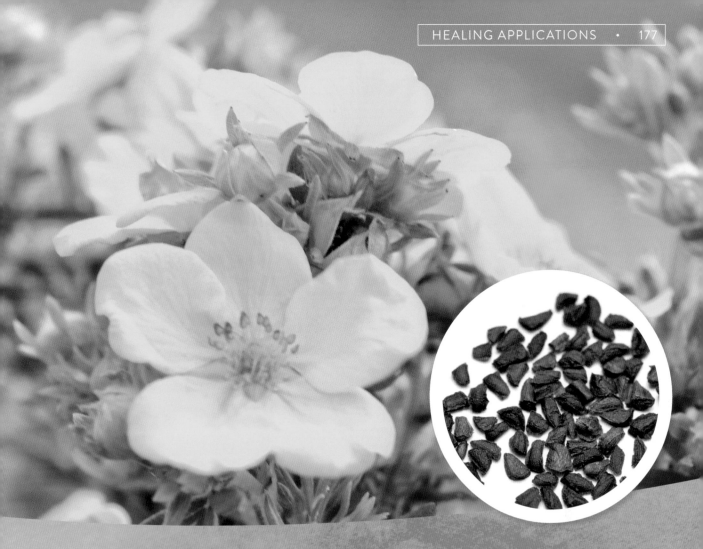

EVENING PRIMROSE OIL

As the name suggests, the bright yellow flowers of the evening primrose bloom at night. The flower probably originated in Mexico and Central America, but it is now found in just about every temperate region of the world. The oil, which is high in omega-3 and omega-6 fatty acids, is derived from the seeds of the evening primrose through cold press extraction.

Research has shown that topical application of fatty acids like omega-3 and omega-6 can reduce inflammation and boost immune system response. This makes evening primrose a great oil to use for those with skin conditions, such as eczema or psoriasis. It can also be rubbed on the hair and scalp to prevent hair loss. When using evening primrose over a large area, it is best to combine it with other carrier oils, such as avocado or grapeseed; but the oil can also be used on its own with a few drops of your favorite essential oil for a soothing facial treatment.

The cold press extraction process used to obtain the oil helps preserve the nutrients that would otherwise be lost if heat were used. Because of this, it is best to store evening primrose oil in the refrigerator after it is opened, to extend its shelf life up to twelve months.

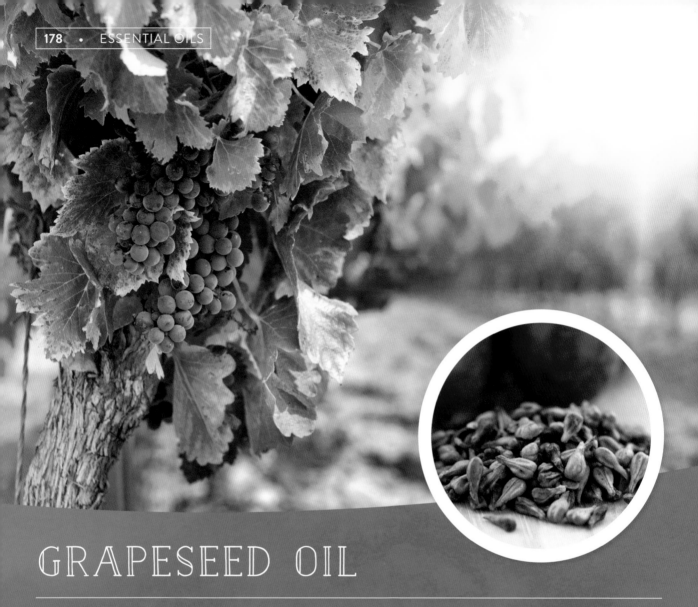

GRAPESEED OIL

Often a byproduct of wine-making, grapeseed oil is pressed from the seeds of grapes. These little seeds are chock-full of antioxidants and nutrients, and the oil that is extracted from them is powerful yet gentle on skin. This has made grapeseed oil a popular addition to many pricey cosmetics, lotions, and sunscreens. But you can buy the oil for a fraction of the price and still reap the benefits!

As a carrier oil, grapeseed is especially helpful for those with sensitive, oily, or acne-prone skin. It has antiseptic and astringent properties, which helps to heal and fight off blemishes. The oil is also loaded with plant compounds called "oligomeric proanthocyanidin complexes," or OPCs. Studies have shown that OPCs have potent antioxidant action, protecting the skin from free radicals and preventing premature aging and wrinkles. And grapeseed oil has plenty of vitamin E, helping to nourish the skin and keep it looking smooth and soft. And as a lighter oil than many others, grapeseed can be used on the skin and hair without leaving behind greasy residue.

Grapeseed has a very light scent, so it mixes well with many essential oils. Be sure to look for an oil that has been cold-pressed and processed without solvents, to ensure you have the purest oil possible.

HAZELNUT OIL

If you've ever enjoyed a spoonful (or two) of chocolate hazelnut spread on your toast, you already know how delicious the nut can be. But the oil extracted from the hazelnut is more than just a culinary delight: with its faint, nutty scent, non-greasy texture, and its benefits to all skin types, hazelnut oil is a great addition to your carrier oil collection.

Known especially for its astringent qualities, hazelnut oil is prized for its use in skin care. In fact, in Turkey—where more than 60 percent of hazelnuts are produced—the oil has been used for hundreds of years as a skin moisturizer and bath oil. Hazelnut is also an excellent oil to use for those with oily skin: although it seems like an oxymoron, hazelnut oil actually helps to balance the oils on the skin, while at the same time having a moisturizing and softening effect.

When refrigerated after opening, hazelnut oil has a shelf life of at least a year, and can last up to two. Since it is a nut oil, be sure to consult a doctor before using if you have any kind of nut allergy.

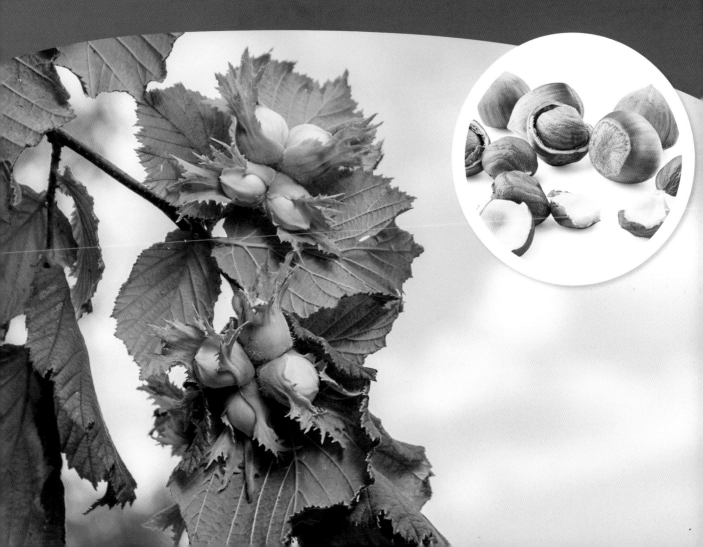

JOJOBA OIL

Native to the Southwestern United States and northern Mexico, jojoba is often grown commercially for its oil—which is actually a liquid wax. The oil has been prized for hundreds of years by Native Americans, who used to heat jojoba seeds to soften them, and then grind them into a salve to soften skin and hair and to treat burns.

Jojoba's unique designation as a wax gives it the property of being more like human sebum—the oil produced by the sebaceous glands in our skin—than any other carrier oil. This makes it an excellent oil to use on the face and neck, or anywhere you'd rather not see the oily "sheen" of a traditional oil. Jojoba is also a natural antifungal, so it works well with essential oils that have antifungal properties. The oil can be used to soothe acne, psoriasis, sunburn, and chapped skin. It may even help to prevent hair loss, by unclogging hair follicles.

Organic, 100 percent jojoba oil is relatively cheap. And like coconut oil, jojoba has a particularly long shelf life, thanks to its very long fatty acid chains and ability to resist oxidation. So don't be afraid to stock up on this amazing oil!

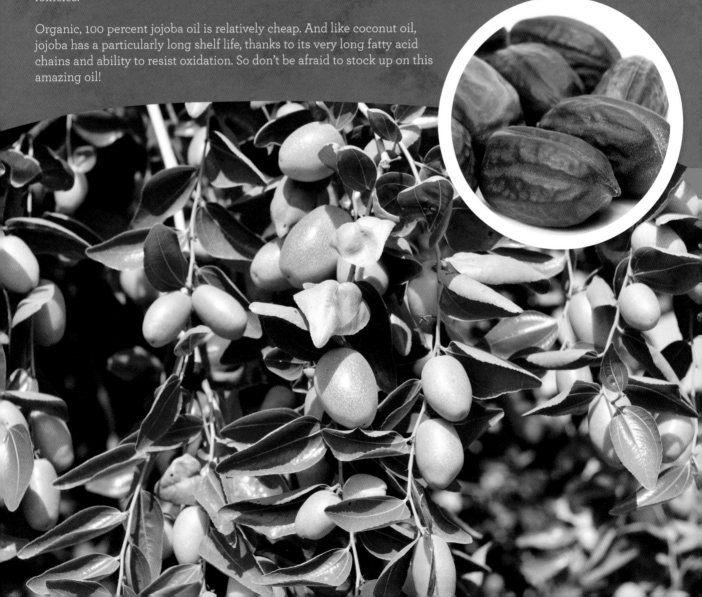

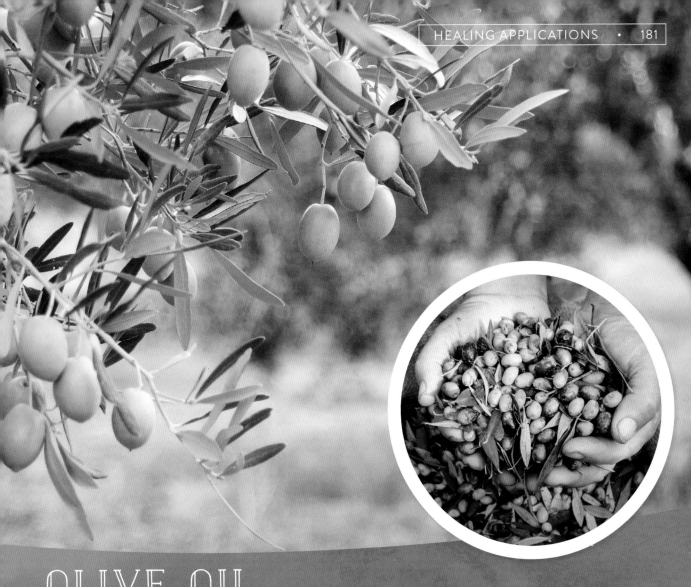

OLIVE OIL

No doubt you've used olive oil in salad dressing, tossed with roasted veggies, or as a dip for Italian bread. But the ubiquitous oil is also great to have on hand to use as a carrier oil. While you may not always have a bottle of avocado or jojoba oil in the pantry, olive oil is so widely used that the odds are good you'll always have some at the ready!

But there are pros and cons to using this popular oil as a carrier oil. For instance, olive oil is readily available, easy to find, and full of omega fatty acids; but it also has a stronger scent than many oils, leaves a greasy feeling on the skin, and has a relatively short shelf life. But it's a great oil to use for those with nut or seed allergies, as so many oils are derived from these possible allergens. And because it's thicker than many carrier oils, it's excellent to use on dry skin.

Be sure to look for extra virgin cold-pressed olive oil, as this extraction process helps to retain all of the vitamins, minerals, and proteins in the oil. Also, steer clear of cheaper brands, which are known to mix olive with less-expensive vegetable oils to cut down on costs.

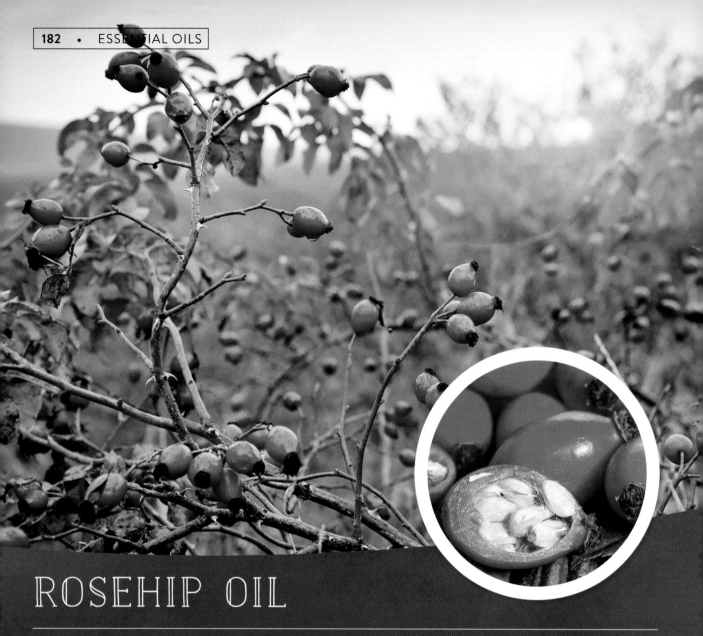

ROSEHIP OIL

Native to the southern Andes in Chile, the wild rose bush provides the seeds from which rosehip seed oil is extracted. Rumor has it the Duchess of Cambridge is fond of this healing oil, which was used by ancient Mayans and Native Americans for its skin-smoothing and healing properties.

Rosehip has enjoyed a surge in popularity in recent years, and for good reason: the oil is high in omega-3 and omega-6 fatty acids, as well as vitamin E and beta-Carotene, which is a form of vitamin A. Studies of the oil have shown it to be effective at reducing wrinkles and sunspots, as well as treating a myriad of skin conditions: scars, sun damage, eczema, psoriasis, dry skin, brittle nails—rosehip oil isn't afraid to tackle them all! The oil works especially well as a carrier oil for any essential oils that you use in your facial care regimen.

The oil can be either solvent extracted or cold-pressed; as with other oils, it's best to buy cold-pressed to ensure you have the purest oil possible. Store the oil in a cool place out of direct light, and use it within a year of opening to prevent rosehip's beneficial fatty acids from going bad.

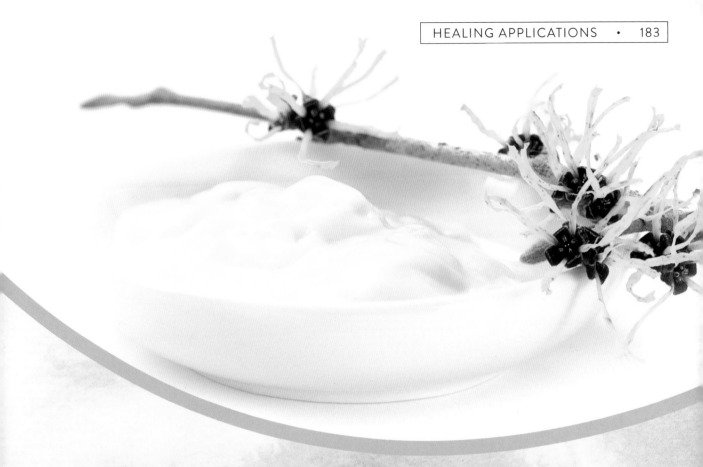

ACNE AND OILY SKIN

Acne may not be a hazard to your health, but it does impair your looks. The problem typically is the result of clogged skin pores. When the pores and follicles (canals that contain hair shafts) are blocked, oil cannot be secreted and builds up. Bacteria feeds on the oil and multiplies. People with oily skin have a greater chance of developing acne, as do teenagers and anyone experiencing hormonal fluctuations. Although not medically proven, stress may also contribute to acne breakouts.

Luckily, quite an array of essential oils are available to help you deal with acne. That's because many oils help manage the specific underlying problems that cause acne: They balance hormones, reduce stress, improve the complexion, and regulate the skin's oil production. This makes aromatherapy the ideal treatment for blemishes, pimples, and other skin eruptions. Commercial acne remedies have long recognized this.

A salt and essential oil compress is a good way to start your acne home care program. For persistent or especially troublesome eruptions, immediately follow the compress with the Intensive Blemish Treatment (both recipes on page 184).

If you have oily skin, use the facial toner (page 184) daily. Or you can choose from any of the skin-drying and antiseptic essential oils from the following list, and then dilute them in a base of witch hazel and aloe vera gel, both of which are readily available at drugstores. The witch hazel contains alcohol, so it is especially drying, and there's no disputing that aloe vera is one of the most beneficial and healing herbs to put on your skin. Combine these with essential oils and prepare yourself for a dazzling complexion!

FACIAL TONER FOR OILY COMPLEXIONS

- 12 drops lemongrass oil
- 6 drops juniper berry oil
- 2 drops ylang ylang oil
- 1 ounce witch hazel lotion
- 1 ounce aloe vera gel

Combine all of the ingredients in a glass bottle. Give the mixture a good shake and it's done! Apply at least once a day. If you find witch hazel too drying, vinegar is an excellent substitute. It is not as drying as the witch hazel and helps to retain the skin's natural acid balance.

ESSENTIAL OILS FOR ACNE OR AN OILY COMPLEXION:

CEDARWOOD	GERANIUM	LEMONGRASS
CLARY SAGE	JUNIPER BERRY	SANDALWOOD
EUCALYPTUS	LAVENDER	TEA TREE
FRANKINCENSE	LEMON	

ZIT ZAP COMPRESS

- 4 drops cedarwood oil
- 2 drops eucalyptus oil
- 1 teaspoon Epsom salts
- 1/4 cup boiling water

Pour the boiling water over the Epsom salts. When the salts are dissolved and the water has cooled just enough to not burn the skin, add the essential oils. Soak a small absorbent cloth in the hot solution, then press the cloth against the blemishes for about one minute. Repeat several times by rewetting the cloth in the same solution.

INTENSIVE BLEMISH TREATMENT

- 12 drops tea tree oil
- 1/2 teaspoon Oregon grape root, powdered
- a few drops of water
- 800 units vitamin E (optional)

Stir the water and oils into the herb powder to make a paste. Apply as a mask directly on the blemished area. Let the paste dry and keep it on your skin for at least 20 minutes, then rinse off. This routine can be done more than once a day, if you wish. The vitamin E can be obtained by poking open a vitamin capsule and squeezing out the oil. It is a good addition when obstinate sores need to heal or if there is any chance of scarring.

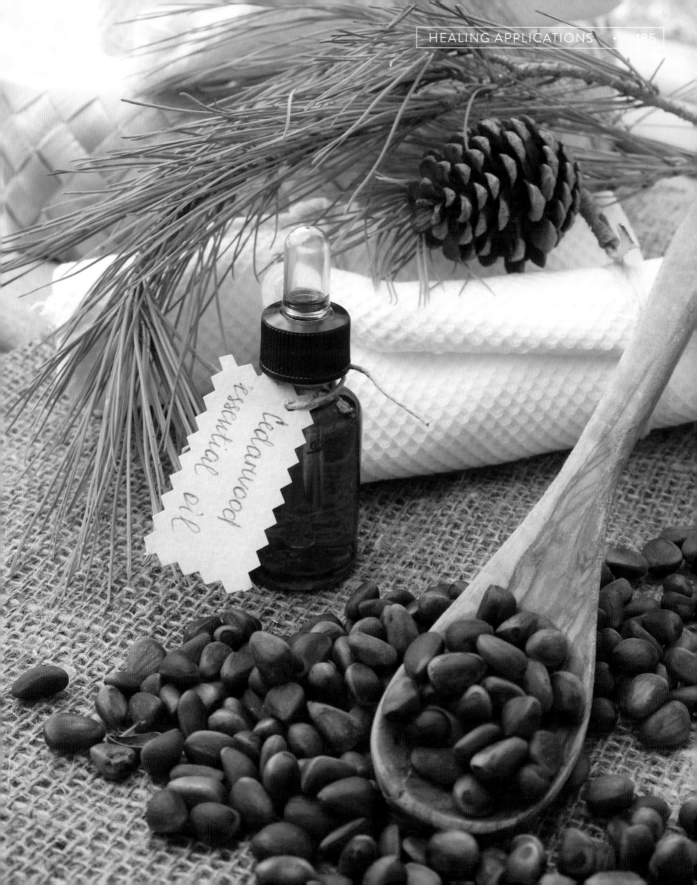

Cedarwood Essential oil

ASTHMA

The characteristic wheezing of asthma is made by the effort to push air through swollen, narrowed bronchial passages. During an asthma attack, stale air cannot be fully exhaled because the bronchioles are swollen and clogged with mucous, and thus less fresh air can be inhaled. The person gasps and labors for breath. Allergic reactions to food, stress, and airborne allergens are the common causes of asthma. Allergies trigger production of histamine, which dilates blood vessels and constricts airways. Asthma sufferers fight an ongoing battle with such low-level congestion, which is actually an attempt by unhappy lungs to rid themselves of irritations.

Many aromatherapy books warn against using essential oils to treat asthma. Some asthmatics are sensitive to fragrance and find that it triggers their attacks. While you certainly don't want to make the situation any worse, aromatherapy offers promising results when used judiciously.

The safest time to try aromatherapy treatments is in between attacks. Use a chest rub made from essential oils that have decongestive and antihistamine properties, such as peppermint and (diluted) ginger. German chamomile, which contains chamazulene, is thought to actually prevent the release of histamine. Frankincense, marjoram, and rose encourage deep breathing and allow lungs to expand. To reduce bronchial spasms, use these relaxants: chamomile, lavender, rose, geranium, and marjoram.

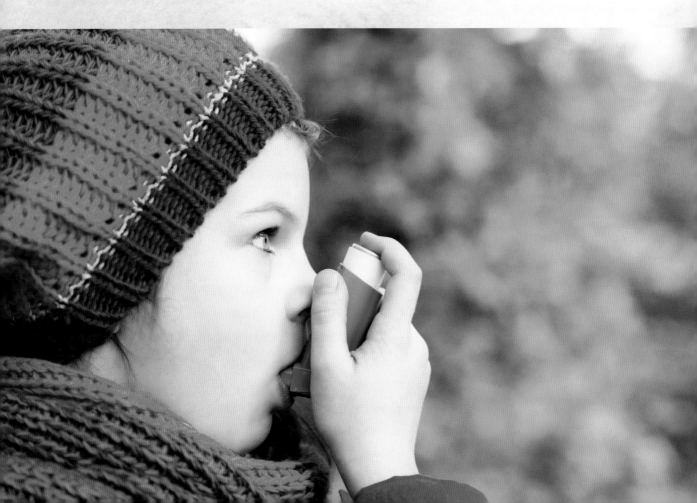

STEAM

A lavender steam can be used by some asthmatics even during an attack. The steam opens airways, while lavender quickly relaxes lung spasms. This may halt the attack right in its tracks or at least make it less severe. As an added bonus, lavender also relaxes the mind, so it helps dissipate the panic you feel when you can't catch your breath.

If you find that steaming only makes it more difficult to breathe, use an aromatherapy diffuser or a humidifier instead. For small children, put some very hot water in the bathtub, add several drops of lavender essential oil, and hold the child in your arms over the steam. You can also rub someone's feet with an aromatherapy massage oil.

Essential oils are not powerful enough to heal an asthmatic condition all by themselves. Herbs that repair lung damage and improve breathing are also needed, along with avoiding whatever sparks the allergic reaction. If this means stress, then other aromatherapy techniques such as massage, relaxation techniques, and fragrant baths can help you de-stress your life.

ESSENTIAL OILS FOR ASTHMA:

CHAMOMILE

EUCALYPTUS (don't use during an attack)

FRANKINCENSE (deepens breathing and allows lungs to expand)

GERANIUM

GINGER

LAVENDER

MARJORAM

PEPPERMINT

ROSE

ASTHMA INHALATION RUB

- 6 drops lavender oil
- 4 drops geranium oil
- 1 drop marjoram oil
- 1 drop peppermint or ginger oil
- 1 ounce carrier oil

Combine the ingredients. Rub on chest as needed, especially before bedtime. Since asthmatics can be extremely sensitive to scent, do a sniff test first. Test the formula by simply sniffing it to make sure there is no adverse reaction.

BLADDER INFECTION

Bladder infections are common, especially in women. So common, in fact, that you may already be familiar with the medical term cystitis to describe the inflammation that can result when bladder infections are unattended. Fortunately, several essential oils can come to the rescue. Juniper berry, sandalwood, chamomile, pine, tea tree, and bergamot are especially effective treatments. However, juniper berry is so strong that it could irritate the kidneys if the bladder infection has spread into them. If that is the case, stick to the other oils. In fact, if there is any chance that you have a kidney infection, be sure to seek a doctor's opinion, as it can have serious consequences.

Apply a massage oil or a compress containing the essential oils listed in the recipe over the bladder, which is located under the lower abdomen, once or twice daily as an adjunct to herbal, nutritional, or even drug treatments.

Added to a bath, these same essential oils can be used during an active infection and will help prevent future infections. If taking a full bath isn't practical, then try a sitz bath.

ESSENTIAL OILS FOR BLADDER INFECTIONS:

BERGAMOT

CEDARWOOD

CYPRESS

FIR

FRANKINCENSE

JUNIPER BERRY (don't use if there's a kidney infection)

SANDALWOOD

TEA TREE

BLADDER INFECTION OIL

- 8 drops juniper berry or cypress oil
- 6 drops tea tree oil
- 6 drops bergamot oil
- 2 drops fennel oil
- 2 ounces carrier oil

Combine the ingredients. Massage over the bladder area once daily. For a preventive treatment, add a tablespoon of this same oil to your bath.

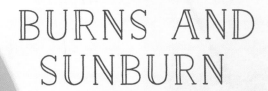

BURNS AND SUNBURN

The first step in treating any minor burn or sunburn is to quickly immerse the afflicted area in cold water (about 50°F) containing a few drops of essential oil. Or you can apply a cold compress that has been soaked in the same water. If the person feels overheated or if the eyelids are sunburned, place the compress on the forehead.

Burned skin is tender to the touch, so spraying a remedy is preferable to dabbing it on. A spray also is extra cooling and is especially handy when sunburn covers a large area.

For your burn wash, compress, or spray, lavender is an all-time favorite among aromatherapists. Lavender and aloe vera juice both promote new cell growth, reduce inflammation, stop infection, and decrease pain. Aloe has even been used successfully on radiation burns. There are several other essential oils that reduce the pain of burns and help them heal, so feel free to experiment. Use them in the same proportions suggested for lavender, except rose oil for which 1 drop equals 5 drops of other essential oils.

VINEGAR

A small amount of vinegar helps to heal a minor burn and provides an additional cooling effect, but it is painful on an open wound. Reserve it for cases in which the skin is unbroken. In general, stick to treating minor, first-degree burns at home, and leave the care of deeper or more extensive burns to a doctor.

ESSENTIAL OILS FOR BURNS AND SUNBURN:

CHAMOMILE	**PEPPERMINT** (cooling in small amounts)
GERANIUM	**ROSE**
LAVENDER	**TEA TREE**
MARJORAM	

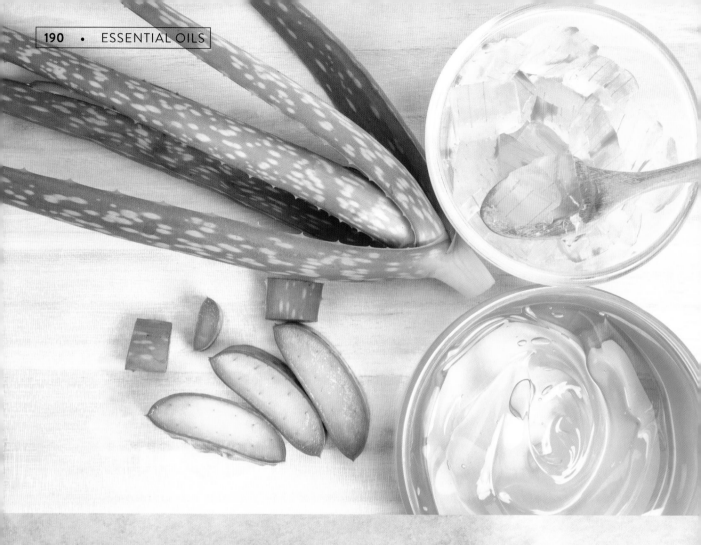

EMERGENCY BURN WASH/COMPRESS

- 5 drops lavender oil
- 1 pint water, about 50°F

Add the essential oil to the water and stir well to disperse the oil. Immerse the burned area for several minutes, or take a soft cloth, soak it in the water, and apply it to the burn. Leave the compress on for several minutes, then resoak and reapply at least twice more.

SUNBURN SOOTHER

- 20 drops lavender oil
- 4 ounces aloe vera juice
- 200 IU vitamin E oil
- 1 tablespoon vinegar

Combine ingredients. Shake well before using. Keep this remedy in a spritzer bottle, and use as often as needed. If you keep the spray in the refrigerator, the coolness will provide extra relief. For the best healing, make sure you use aloe vera juice and not drugstore gel. Apply as often as possible until you are healed.

CONGESTION, SINUS, AND LUNG

The most common cause of sinus and lung congestion is a cold or flu virus. Additionally, secondary bacterial infections that follow on the heels of colds and flus can be especially nasty, irritating the delicate lining in the respiratory tract. The mucous that causes the congestion is produced to protect that lining and wash away the infection.

For quick relief, thin out congestion by using the essential oils of eucalyptus, peppermint, and bergamot combined with steam. Remember how much easier it is to breath when you step into a steamy, hot shower? The steam opens up tightened bronchial passages, allowing the essential oils to penetrate and wipe out the viral or bacterial infection that is causing the problem.

Two of the best essential oils to eliminate infection are lavender and eucalyptus. In fact, studies prove that a two percent dilution of eucalyptus oil kills 70 percent of airborne staphylococcus bacteria. Anise, peppermint, and eucalyptus reduce coughing, perhaps by suppressing the brain's cough reflex. Cypress dries a persistently runny nose.

A vapor balm (a salve containing essential oils) or massage oil can be rubbed over the chest, back, and throat to relieve congestion. Vapor balms increase circulation and warmth in the chest as they are absorbed through the skin. Placing a flannel cloth on the chest after rubbing in the oil will increase the warming action. Commercial products, such as Vicks VapoRub, still use derivatives of essential oils (or their synthetic oil counterparts) such as thymol from thyme and menthol from mint, in a petroleum ointment base, but more natural alternatives are available from your health store. Essential oil molecules are also easily inhaled from the balm.

THERAPEUTIC STEAM

To create a therapeutic steam, add a few drops of essential oil to a pan of water that is simmering on the stove. You can also use a humidifier—some actually provide a compartment for essential oils. If you are at the office or traveling and steaming is impractical, try inhaling a tissue scented with the oils, or use a natural nasal inhaler. These are available in health stores and are found online, or you can make your own. If you don't have a diffuser but would like to disinfect the air, simply combine water and essential oils and dispense the solution from a spray bottle.

The steam recipe given here uses eucalyptus, which is simple and effective, but you can replace it with other essential oils. If you are having trouble deciding which oils to use, refer to the essential oil profiles to determine their differences and which oil might have additional qualities that you would like to include.

ESSENTIAL OIL STEAM

- 1/4 teaspoon eucalyptus oil
- 3 cups of water

Bring water to a simmer, turn off heat, and add essential oils. Set the pan where you can sit down next to it. Place your face over the steam and drape a towel over the back of your head to form a mini-sauna. Breathe in the steam, coming out for fresh air as needed. Do at least three rounds of steam inhalation several times a day. Fresh or dried eucalyptus leaves can be added to the water instead of the pure essential oil. Whichever essential oil you use, be sure to keep your eyes closed while steaming. It's okay to use this steam as often as you like.

NASAL INHALER

- 5 drops eucalyptus oil
- 1/4 teaspoon coarse salt

Place the salt in a small vial (glass is best) with a tight lid and add essential oil. The salt will absorb the oil so it won't spill when you carry it. When needed, open the vial and inhale deeply. This same technique can be used with any essential oil listed above. Sniff as needed throughout the day.

VAPOR RUB

- 12 drops eucalyptus oil
- 5 drops peppermint oil
- 5 drops thyme oil
- 1 ounce olive oil

Combine ingredients in a glass bottle. Shake well to mix oils evenly. Gently massage into chest and throat. Use one to five times per day and especially just before bed.

ESSENTIAL OILS FOR FIGHTING RESPIRATORY INFECTIONS:

BENZOIN	MARJORAM
CLOVE	TEA TREE
EUCALYPTUS	THYME
LAVENDER	

ESSENTIAL OILS TO EASE MUCOUS CONGESTION:

BENZOIN	EUCALYPTUS
BIRCH	GINGER
CEDARWOOD	PEPPERMINT
CLOVE	TEA TREE
CYPRESS	THYME

CUTS, SCRAPES, AND BRUISES

Simple cuts and scrapes can easily be treated with antiseptic essential oils. A mist of diluted oil is an excellent way to apply them. Herbal salves containing antiseptic essential oils are also effective in treating scrapes or wounds that aren't too deep. Need to protect your cut? Many of the resins and balsams such as benzoin, frankincense, and myrrh actually form a protective barrier over the wound that acts as an antiseptic "Band-Aid." In an emergency, don't forget that you can dab a little lavender or tea tree oil directly on a scrape as they are among the least irritating of oils.

ESSENTIAL OILS FOR CUTS AND SCRAPES:

BENZOIN	GERANIUM	MYRRH
EUCALYPTUS	LAVENDER	ROSE
FRANKINCENSE	LEMON	TEA TREE

GERM FIGHTER SPRAY

- 12 drops tea tree oil
- 6 drops eucalyptus oil
- 6 drops lemon oil
- 2 ounces distilled water or herbal tincture

Combine the ingredients and shake well to disperse the oils before each use. Dispense this formula from a spray bottle as needed on minor cuts, burns, or abrasions to prevent infection and speed healing. As an alternative to the distilled water, you can use a tincture made from an antiseptic herb such as Oregon grape root. If you do this, keep in mind that tinctures contain alcohol, which will make the essential oils disperse better and increase the antiseptic properties of the spray, but it will also sting more on an open wound. Apply immediately and then several times a day to keep the wound clean and encourage healing.

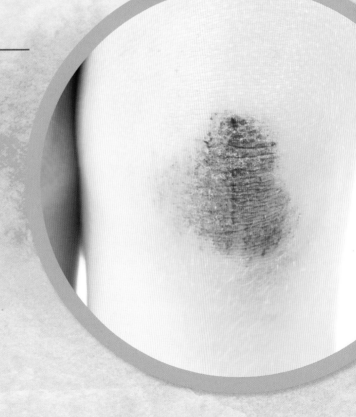

DEPRESSION/ANXIETY

It's no secret that fragrance lifts and enhances one's mood. The aroma of many plants, such as the elegant orange blossom aroma of neroli or the closely related and less expensive petitgrain, as well as jasmine, sandalwood, and ylang ylang, relieve depression and anxiety. Modern aromatherapists agree with the seventeenth-century herbalist John Gerard, who recommended the use of clary sage to ease depression, paranoia, mental fatigue, and nervous disorders. Researchers at International Flavors and Fragrances, Inc., in New Jersey have found that orange reduces anxiety. East Indians traditionally use basil to prevent agitation and nightmares.

Fragrances are generally effective for people who have mild forms of depression that do not require drugs. And they can be especially helpful when the doctor is trying to wean patients off drugs. Aromatherapy can be used safely in conjunction with antidepressant medications because it will not interfere with the dosage or effect. If you are currently taking prescription drugs to deal with depression or anxiety, however, don't abruptly stop taking them or replace them with essential oils without your doctor's okay.

Massage and bath oils are probably the most relaxing forms of antidepressant aromatherapy. If you wish to make your environment more uplifting at home or at work, try using an aromatherapy room spray, or put the essential oils in an aromatherapy diffuser, potpourri cooker, or a pan of simmering water. You can make a constant companion of your favorite oil, or of a blend of oils, by carrying them in a small vial. Then, when you need a lift, just take a whiff.

ESSENTIAL OILS FOR RELIEVING ANXIETY AND DEPRESSION:

BERGAMOT	CYPRESS	LEMON	SANDALWOOD
CEDARWOOD	GERANIUM	MARJORAM	ROSE
CINNAMON	JASMINE	NEROLI	YLANG YLANG
CLARY SAGE	LAVENDER	ORANGE	

UPLIFTING FORMULA 1

- 6 drops bergamot oil
- 3 drops petitgrain oil
- 3 drops geranium oil
- 1 drop neroli (expensive, so optional)
- 2 ounces carrier oil

Combine all the ingredients. Use as a massage oil, add 1 or 2 teaspoons to your bath, or add 1 teaspoon to a foot bath. For an equally uplifting room or facial spritzer, substitute the same amount of water for the carrier oil in this formula. Put the water formula in a spray bottle, and spritz or sniff throughout the day as needed.

UPLIFTING FORMULA 2

- 4 drops frankincense oil
- 4 drops jasmine oil
- 2 drops lemon oil
- 2 ounces carrier oil

Combine all ingredients and use as suggested in Uplifting Formula 1.

UPLIFTING FORMULA 3

- 7 drops bergamot oil
- 4 drops vetiver oil
- 3 drops clary sage oil
- 2 ounces carrier oil

Combine all ingredients and use as suggested in Uplifting Formula 1.

ANXIETY-REDUCING FORMULA 1

- 7 drops sandalwood oil
- 4 drops bergamot oil
- 4 drops rose oil
- 3 drops orange oil
- 2 ounces carrier oil

Combine all ingredients and use as suggested in Uplifting Formula 1.

ANXIETY-REDUCING FORMULA 2

- 10 drops bergamot oil
- 4 drops lavender oil
- 4 drops Roman chamomile oil
- 2 ounces carrier oil

Combine all ingredients and use as suggested in Uplifting Formula 1.

DERMATITIS, PSORIASIS, AND ECZEMA

Dermatitis is an inflammation of the skin that causes itching, redness, and skin lesions. It's difficult even for dermatologists to uncover the source of this bothersome skin problem. Some obvious causes, though, are contact with an irritant such as poison oak or ivy, harsh chemicals, or anything to which one is allergic. Stress also seems to be a contributing factor in many types of dermatitis. Essential oils that counter stress, soothe inflammation and itching, soften roughness, and are both antiseptic and drying are used to treat these skin conditions.

One type of dermatitis is eczema, a word that describes a series of symptoms rather than a disease. Eczema is characterized by crusty, oozing skin that itches and may feel like it burns. Psoriasis is a dermatitis with red lesions covered by silver-like scales that flake off. This condition can be hereditary, but its cause is unknown. It has an annoying tendency to come and go for no apparent reason.

One of the best vehicles for essential oils in these cases is an herbal salve that already contains a base of skin-healing herbs such as comfrey and calendula. You can use a store-bought herbal salve or one that you make yourself. Stir in 15 drops (or less) of essential oils per ounce of salve. Since salves come in a two-ounce jar, that means adding no more than 30 drops; use less if the salve already contains some essential oils.

Secondary skin infections, which often occur with eczema, need to be treated with antiseptic essential oils, such as those suggested for acne.

ESSENTIAL OILS FOR DERMATITIS:

BIRCH	PEPPERMINT (for itching)
CHAMOMILE	ROSEMARY
LAVENDER	TEA TREE

DERMATITIS SKIN CARE

- 8 drops tea tree oil
- 8 drops chamomile oil
- 1 teaspoon Oregon grape tincture
- 2 ounces healing salve

With a toothpick, stir the tincture and essential oils into the salve. This will make the salve semi-liquid. Apply one to four times a day.

DIAPER RASH

Aromatherapy baby oil and powder can help protect your little ones from diaper rash. The oil repels moisture, and the powder absorbs moisture and prevents chafing. Use one or the other with every diaper change, or more often if needed. Baby oil is also good for the skin. Make your own baby powder from plain old corn starch and essential oils.

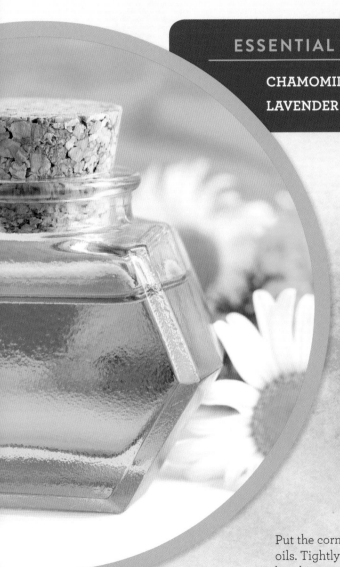

ESSENTIAL OILS FOR DIAPER RASH:

CHAMOMILE   SANDALWOOD

LAVENDER   TEA TREE

AROMATHERAPY BABY OIL

- 6 drops lavender oil
- 2 drops chamomile oil
- 2 ounces carrier oil

Combine the ingredients. Use after each diaper change and as an all-over massage oil. The same amount of lavender and chamomile can also be stirred into a basic herbal salve with a toothpick and used on the diaper area.

FRAGRANT BABY POWDER

- 20 drops (1/4 teaspoon) lavender oil
- 5 drops mandarin or tangerine oil
- 1/2 pound corn starch

Put the corn starch in a plastic zip-lock bag and drop in the essential oils. Tightly close the bag, and toss back and forth to distribute the oil, breaking up any clumps by pressing them with your fingers through the bag. Let stand at least four days to distribute the essential oil. Spice, salt, or Parmesan cheese shakers with large holes in their lids make good powder applicators. Powder after each diaper change or bath.

DRY SKIN

A dry skin condition can mean rough, cracked hands and a flaky complexion that could eventually lead to excessive wrinkling. Skin conditions like psoriasis and eczema often go hand in hand with dry skin.

For any dry skin product, choose essential oils that balance the production of oil on the skin and also are anti-inflammatory so that they'll reduce irritation and its characteristic puffiness. If your dry skin is also mature skin, the historic "anti-aging" essential oils lavender, geranium, neroli, rosemary, and rose are particularly suitable. These essential oils are also thought to rejuvenate skin by encouraging new cell growth. Other excellent oils to use on dry skin are frankincense, myrrh, and sandalwood. Perhaps their skin rejuvenating characteristics are the reason they have been so highly valued over the last two thousand years!

In small amounts, peppermint increases the production of oil in the skin. Chamomile, carrot seed, and helichrysum reduce inflammation that can accompany dry skin conditions. The latter two even help get rid of precancerous skin conditions that usually appear as raised discolorations on areas most exposed to the sun, such as the hands and face.

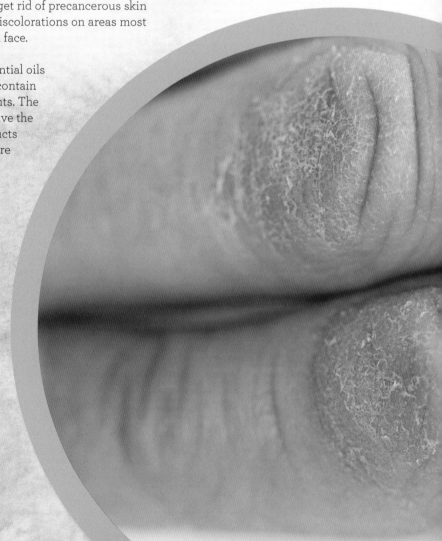

The best way to treat dry skin is with essential oils added to a cream or lotion. Both of these contain water, not just oil as in salves and ointments. The water is absorbed by the skin to help resolve the dryness. Meanwhile, the oil in these products acts as a protective barrier to keep moisture from evaporating out of the skin. Try to purchase as pure a cream as possible. You may even be able to find a cream that already contains essential oils that are good for your dry complexion. If not, purchase an unscented cream, and stir the oils into it yourself. One more thing that you can do for dry skin is to avoid soap, except when your face is honestly dirty. Instead, a gentle oatmeal scrub combined with essential oils should be sufficient.

ESSENTIAL OILS TO PREVENT AGING:

GERANIUM   ROSE

LAVENDER   ROSEMARY

NEROLI

ESSENTIAL OILS FOR DRY SKIN: ALL THE ABOVE OILS PLUS:

FRANKINCENSE   MYRRH   SANDALWOOD

ESSENTIAL OIL TO MOISTURIZE SKIN:

PEPPERMINT

ESSENTIAL OILS FOR REDUCING INFLAMMATION AND PUFFINESS:

CHAMOMILE   LAVENDER

ANTI-AGING COMPLEXION CREAM

- 15 drops geranium oil
- 3 drops rose oil
- 2 drops frankincense or neroli oil
- 2 ounces complexion cream

Stir the essential oils into the cream. Use daily.

DRY COMPLEXION SCRUB

- 6 drops lavender oil
- 2 drops peppermint oil
- 1 tablespoon dried flowers of elder, lavender, or chamomile (optional)
- 2 tablespoons oatmeal
- 1 tablespoon cornmeal

Grind dry ingredients in a blender or electric coffee grinder. (You may also want to consider colloidal oatmeal, which needs no grinding.) Add the essential oils, and stir to distribute. Store in a closed container, and use instead of soap for cleansing your face. For clean skin, moisten 1 teaspoon with enough water to make a paste, dampen your face with a little water, then gently apply scrub. Rinse with warm water. Use this daily instead of soap.

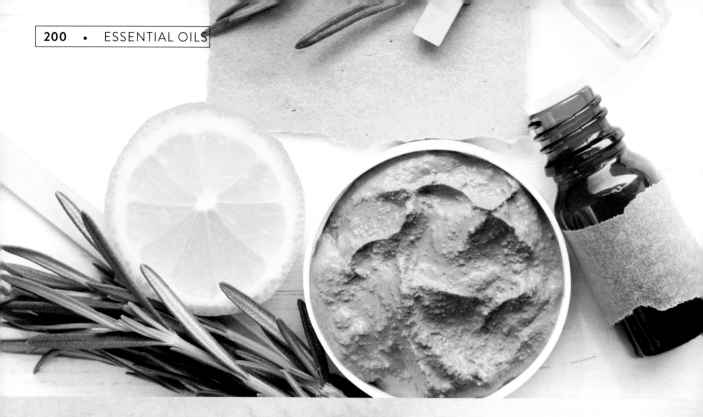

DRY FACIAL SKIN CLAY MASK

- 5 drops lavender oil
- 2 drops geranium oil
- 1 drop helichrysum oil

- 1 drop patchouli oil
- 1 tsp olive oil
- 1 cup cosmetic clay

Blend all ingredients thoroughly. Apply to problem areas of face. Allow to dry for 20 minutes. Wash off with warm water.

WINTER'S DAY HAND LOTION

- 5 drops helichrysum oil
- 5 drops myrrh oil
- 4 drops palmarosa oil
- 4 drops German chamomile oil

- 2 drops carrot seed oil
- 1 drop patchouli oil
- 1 ounce unscented lotion

Blend all ingredients together. Use on hands when they become dry or chapped.

CRACKED HEEL RESCUE FORMULA

- 10 drops frankincense oil
- 10 drops helichrysum oil
- 8 drops lavender oil
- 8 drops tea tree oil

- 5 drops peppermint oil
- 1/2 cup coconut oil
- 1/4 cup beeswax
- 1/4 cup shea butter

Shave and melt the beeswax in coconut oil on stove. Add shea butter and allow the mixture to cool until you can comfortably stir it with your finger. Add remaining ingredients and stir thoroughly. Use liberally on cracked feet. Cover your feet with socks to prevent oil stains.

EARACHE

An earache is most likely due to an infection. While this is not the sort of condition to treat exclusively with aromatherapy, an aromatherapy massage oil rubbed on the outside of the ear is an excellent adjunct to other treatments. Dilute an antiseptic essential oil like lavender or tea tree in olive oil. Lavender has the added benefit of helping to reduce inflammation. Gently rub this around the outside of the ear and down along the lymph nodes on the side of the neck. Do not put it in the ear itself. Instead, make a warm compress using these same oils and place it directly over the ear. Always treat both ears, even if only one hurts, and continue treating them for a couple days after the pain is gone.

Basil and helichrysum are mild enough to apply neat. Simply dampen a cotton ball and apply a drop of either oil. Place gently in your affected ear (don't force or push it in). Use as long as needed.

ESSENTIAL OILS FOR EARACHE:

BASIL	LAVENDER
HELICHRYSUM	TEA TREE

EAR RUB FORMULA

- 3 drops lavender oil
- 3 drops tea tree oil
- 1 tablespoon carrier oil

Combine ingredients. Rub this oil around the ear and down the side of the neck. For children, remember to use half this dilution (no more than 3 drops total of essential oil to 1 tablespoon carrier oil). Rub on two to four times a day, especially before bed.

COTTON BALL BLEND FORMULA

- 1 drop basil oil
- 1 drop frankincense oil
- 1 drop lavender oil
- 1 drop tea tree oil
- 1 tablespoon carrier oil

Combine all ingredients. Saturate a cotton ball with the blend and place it gently inside the ear. Use as long as needed.

EYESTRAIN/INFLAMMATION

Eyestrain is common in this age of proliferating computer screens and mobile devices. Of course, essential oils should never go directly into the eye, even when diluted. However, you can ease eye discomfort with either a cold or warm compress. For most eye problems such as sties or inflammation, use essential oils such as lavender or chamomile because they will reduce the swelling.

For eyestrain, use a warm compress. To reduce inflammation, including that early morning eye puffiness, try using a cold compress. If you have the time, relax with the compress on your eyes for at least five minutes, although even a couple of minutes will provide some benefit.

A quick treatment for eyestrain that is especially handy when traveling is to use chamomile tea bags. Since the smell of chamomile is soothing and relaxing, too, you will receive an additional aromatherapy treatment to relieve the stress of the road.

ESSENTIAL OILS FOR EYESTRAIN AND INFLAMMATION:

CHAMOMILE

LAVENDER

EYE TEA

- 2 bags of chamomile tea

Steep the tea bags for a few minutes in a couple tablespoons of hot water, as if making a very strong tea. Let cool just enough so that it is comfortable for a warm treatment or cool at least to room temperature for a cool treatment. Lie down and place a tea bag over each eye, then cover with a soft cloth. Use as often as you like.

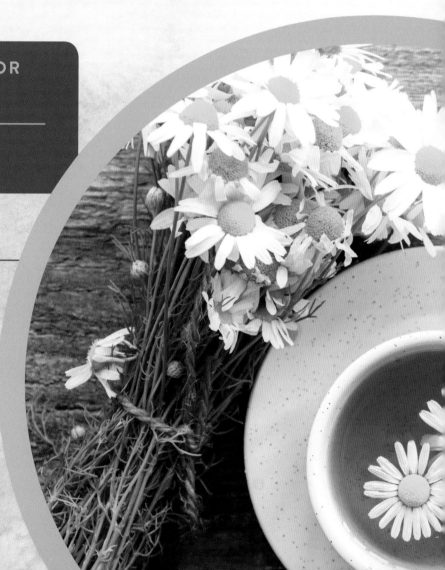

FATIGUE

Just as some aromas calm you down, others will perk you up. Researchers found that this is especially true of eucalyptus and pine. The spicy aromas of clove, basil, black pepper, and cinnamon—and to a lesser degree patchouli, lemongrass, and sage—are other aromatherapy stimulants that reduce drowsiness, irritability, and headaches. Some large companies have experimented with circulating lemon, cypress, and peppermint through their air-conditioning and heating systems to keep employees alert. These stimulating essential oils have been shown to prevent the sharp drop in attention that typically hits after working for thirty minutes. Clove, cinnamon, lemon, cardamom, fennel, and angelica act as stimulants. Using aromatherapy stimulants is healthier for you than ingesting stimulants such as coffee because the scents provide energy without causing an adrenaline rush that strains the adrenal glands.

ESSENTIAL OILS FOR ENERGY:

CINNAMON	FIR	PEPPERMINT
CLOVE	GINGER	ROSEMARY
CYPRESS	LEMON	
EUCALYPTUS	LEMONGRASS	

PICK-ME-UP COMBO

- 8 drops lemon oil
- 2 drops eucalyptus oil
- 2 drops peppermint oil
- 1 drop cinnamon leaf oil
- 1 drop cardamom oil
- 2 ounces carrier oil

Combine the ingredients. Use as a massage oil, add 2 teaspoons to your bath, or add 1 teaspoon to a footbath. Without the carrier oil, this combination can be used in an aromatherapy diffuser, simmering pan of water, or a potpourri cooker, or it can be added to 2 ounces of water for an air spray. The cardamom oil is optional, but, oh, does it enhance this massage oil! Use it as often as you like.

ENERGIZING MASSAGE COMBO

- 10 drops eucalyptus oil
- 10 drops rosemary oil
- 5 drops cypress oil
- 3 drops juniper oil
- 3 drops spruce oil
- 2 tablespoons carrier oil

Combine the ingredients. Use as a massage oil, add 2 teaspoons to your bath, or add 1 teaspoon to a footbath.

MORNING KICK-STARTER BLEND

- 20 drops rosemary
- 18 drops elemi oil
- 14 drops basil oil
- 14 drops peppermint oil
- 6 drops ginger oil

Combine all ingredients in a small glass bottle. When you need a jolt of positive energy to get you going, shake the bottle and take a few whiffs.

PURELY POSITIVE BLEND

- 20 drops lime oil
- 20 drops lemon oil
- 15 drops grapefruit oil
- 15 drops peppermint oil
- 15 drops rosemary oil

Combine all ingredients in a small glass bottle. Shake well and smell when you need to beat back fatigue.

KEEP CALM AND STAY STRONG BLEND

- 20 drops cedarwood oil
- 15 drops bergamot oil
- 15 drops geranium oil
- 15 drops lavender oil
- 10 drops sandalwood oil
- 10 drops chamomile oil

Combine all ingredients in a small glass bottle. When needed, shake well and smell. This fortifying blend will brace you for the task at hand, without overdoing it.

FUNGAL INFECTION/ ATHLETE'S FOOT

Many different fungal infections appear on the skin, and the following treatments can often wipe them out. Most people are familiar with ringworm, especially athlete's foot because it is so common. Athlete's foot is so common because feet sweat and then are cloistered in socks and shoes. This creates the moist environment that fungi really love. If sweating feet are part of the problem, you can use sage to decrease perspiration. Peppermint will help relieve the itching that accompanies a fungal infection. Incorporating the essential oils into a cornstarch powder or a vinegar-based preparation will discourage fungal growth because both are quite drying. Vinegar has the extra benefit of destroying fungal infections.

Some of the most effective antifungal essential oils are tea tree and eucalyptus; lemon eucalyptus is particularly helpful. Lavender, myrrh, and geranium are close seconds. A small amount of peppermint essential oil relieves the itching, and since it stimulates blood circulation, it helps perk you up after a long day on your feet. Don't hesitate to use the same essential oils to treat funguses that creep under nails or affect other parts of the body.

An aromatic foot bath is a great way to treat fungal conditions like athlete's foot or to simply revitalize feet after a long day. You simply can't ask for a better way to take your medicine! If you think you don't have time for such a luxury, why not haul the basin in front of the TV, or catch up on your reading while enjoying your soak? Get yourself a basin large enough to accommodate both feet comfortably, fill it with warm water, and add several drops of essential oil. Add Epsom salts to relax tight muscles and soreness.

For a complete anti-fungal treatment, start off with a foot bath, hand soak, or wash that covers the afflicted area. Afterward, dry off thoroughly, then apply the Fungal Fighter Solution with vinegar followed by the Fungal Fighter Powder (page 206). Do the entire routine at least once a day, and apply either the vinegar or the powder a few extra times.

ESSENTIAL OILS FOR FUNGAL INFECTION:

BENZOIN	LEMONGRASS
CLOVE	MYRRH
EUCALYPTUS (especially lemon eucalyptus)	PEPPERMINT
	SANDALWOOD
GERANIUM	TEA TREE
LAVENDER	THYME

AROMATIC FOOT BATH

- 6 drops tea tree oil
- 4 drops sage oil
- 2 drops peppermint oil
- 1–2 quarts water
- 1/4 cup Epsom salts (optional)

Fill a container that is big enough for both feet with very warm water. Add the essential oils, and soak your feet for at least 15 minutes. The Epsom salts are a good addition if your feet are sore or just plain "dog tired." When making any type of foot bath, you can also add a drop of your own choice of essential oil for whatever emotional impact you need. For example, the peppermint suggested in this recipe is an emotional and physical pick-me-up. It feels great at the end of the day, every day, or at least twice a week.

FUNGAL FIGHTER SOLUTION

- 12 drops tea tree oil
- 8 drops geranium oil
- 3 drops thyme oil
- 2 drops myrrh oil
  (expensive, so optional)
- 1 tablespoon tincture of benzoin
- 2 ounces apple cider vinegar

Combine the ingredients, and shake well before each use. Dab this solution on the afflicted area, or use it as a wash at least once a day—more often if possible. You can purchase tincture of benzoin at any drugstore.

FUNGAL FIGHTER POWDER

- 14 drops lemon eucalyptus or
  tea tree oil
- 8 drops geranium oil
- 5 drops sage oil
- 1 drop peppermint oil
- 1/4 cup cornstarch

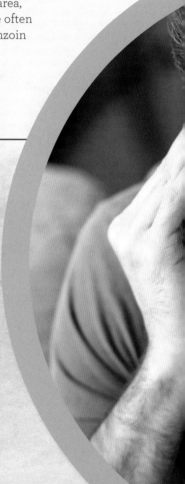

Place the cornstarch in a resealable plastic bag. Sprinkle in the essential oils slowly, trying to distribute them evenly through the powder. Close the bag and toss the powder, breaking up any clumps that form. For long-term storage, keep the powder in a sealed plastic bag or glass or ceramic container, although you probably will find a shake bottle with a perforated lid more convenient to dispense it. A variety of these are sold in housewares departments for the kitchen. Use at least once a day, more often if possible.

HEADACHE

Aromatherapy really proves its worth with headaches. Peppermint, eucalyptus, and lavender are especially helpful in reducing headache pain. A tincture of lavender called "Palsy Drops" was recognized by the British Pharmacopoeia for more than 200 years and was used by physicians to relieve muscle spasms, nervousness, and headaches until the 1940s, when herbs and aroma preparations fell out of favor and new pharmaceuticals became more popular.

Most people find that their headaches respond best to a cold compress, but you can use a warm or hot compress—or alternate the two—for the result that works best. You can also place a second compress at the back of the neck. When you do not have time for compresses, dab a small drop of lavender, eucalyptus, or peppermint oil on each temple. For some people, a hot bath only makes their head pound more. However, if bathing does ease your pain, add a few drops of relaxing lavender or chamomile to your bath water.

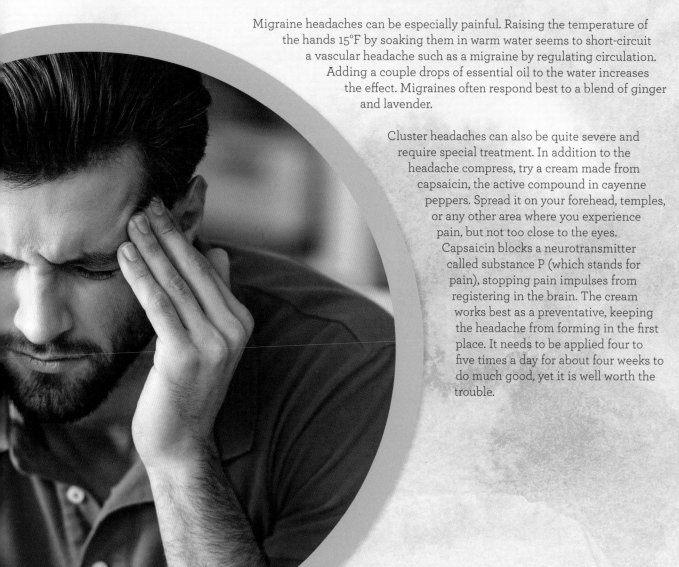

Migraine headaches can be especially painful. Raising the temperature of the hands 15°F by soaking them in warm water seems to short-circuit a vascular headache such as a migraine by regulating circulation. Adding a couple drops of essential oil to the water increases the effect. Migraines often respond best to a blend of ginger and lavender.

Cluster headaches can also be quite severe and require special treatment. In addition to the headache compress, try a cream made from capsaicin, the active compound in cayenne peppers. Spread it on your forehead, temples, or any other area where you experience pain, but not too close to the eyes. Capsaicin blocks a neurotransmitter called substance P (which stands for pain), stopping pain impulses from registering in the brain. The cream works best as a preventative, keeping the headache from forming in the first place. It needs to be applied four to five times a day for about four weeks to do much good, yet it is well worth the trouble.

ESSENTIAL OILS FOR HEADACHES:

BASIL	EUCALYPTUS	LEMONGRASS	ROSEMARY
CHAMOMILE	GINGER	MARJORAM	SPEARMINT
CINNAMON	JASMINE	PATCHOULI	
CLOVE	LAVENDER	PEPPERMINT	

In a 1994 U.S. study by H. Gobel, the essential oils of peppermint and eucalyptus relaxed both the mind and muscles of headache sufferers when the oils were diluted in alcohol and rubbed on their foreheads. Essential oils also can be used to make a compress to place on your forehead whenever a headache hits.

HEADACHE-BE-GONE COMPRESS

- 5 drops lavender or eucalyptus oil
- 1 cup cold water

Add essential oil to water, and swish a soft cloth in it. Wring out the cloth, lie down, and close your eyes. Place the cloth over your forehead and eyes. Use throughout the day, as often as you can.

MIGRAINE HEADACHE HAND SOAK

- 5 drops lavender oil
- 5 drops ginger oil
- 1 quart hot water, about 110°F

Add essential oils to the hot water, and soak hands for at least 3 minutes. This therapy can be done repeatedly.

SOOTHING TEMPLE MASSAGE

- 2 drops eucalyptus oil
- 2 drops lavender oil
- 2 drops spearmint oil
- 2 teaspoons carrier oil

Combine all ingredients. Gently massage mixture over temples and afflicted areas of the head, as well as the neck and shoulders.

HEADACHE STEAM RELIEF

- 2 drops bergamot oil
- 2 drops clary sage oil
- 2 drops marjoram oil
- 1 drop black pepper oil

Add drops to small pot of water and heat on stove. Remove from heat and lean over pot, breathing in deeply.

TENSION-EASING BATH BLEND

- 5 drops eucalyptus oil
- 5 drops Roman chamomile oil
- 5 drops rosemary oil
- 1/2 cup Epsom salts

Fill bath with hot water at the temperature you're comfortable with. Add all ingredients to bath and relax in the tub for as long as desired.

MIGRAINE MASSAGE BLEND

- 2 drops basil oil
- 2 drops lavender oil
- 2 drops marjoram oil
- 2 drops peppermint oil
- 2 drops Roman chamomile
- 3 teaspoons carrier oil

Combine all ingredients. Gently massage mixture over temples and afflicted areas of the head, as well as the neck and shoulders.

RESTFUL HEADACHE PILLOW

- 12 drops lavender oil
- 12 drops marjoram oil
- 1 cup flax seeds
- 8 1/2" x 9" piece of silk cloth

Add the essential oils to flax seeds in a glass jar and let them sit for a week until the oils are absorbed. Fold and stitch the cloth (an old scarf works fine) into a bag measuring approximately 4" x 8 1/2" and add the scented flax seeds. Sew up the opening. Lie down, and lay this "pillow" over your eyes when you feel a headache coming on. Store the pillow in a glass jar to preserve the scent. If the scent starts to dissipate, you can add more essential oil directly through the silk as needed.

HERPES

Herpes is a painful viral infection that appears on the genitals or around the mouth in the form of fever blisters. The herpes virus can lay dormant in the nervous system for a long time, appearing only now and then. Current conventional medicine has little to offer to treat herpes and does not know how to completely eliminate the virus. The virus reactivates when the immune system is weakened, such as when you are under emotional or physical stress. Consider using aromatherapy and other methods to build up your immune system and to relax.

Research shows that creams made from capsaicin, a compound found in cayenne, will deaden the pain of herpes and shingles. The essential oils of cayenne will also work if added to a cream or oil base, but extremely careful with it since too much of this oil can burn the skin. Small amounts of peppermint sometimes also diminish the nerve-tingling pain of herpes and shingles.

Tea tree, especially the type known as niaouli, is the favorite essential oil to treat herpes. Although much more expensive, an essential oil of myrrh is also very effective. Dilute the essential oil of your choice in an equal amount of carrier oil or alcohol, and apply it directly to the herpes blisters. If applied as soon as the blisters begin to appear, any of these oils may prevent it from breaking out. This formula can be used on another virus related to herpes, called herpes zoster, which causes chicken pox and shingles.

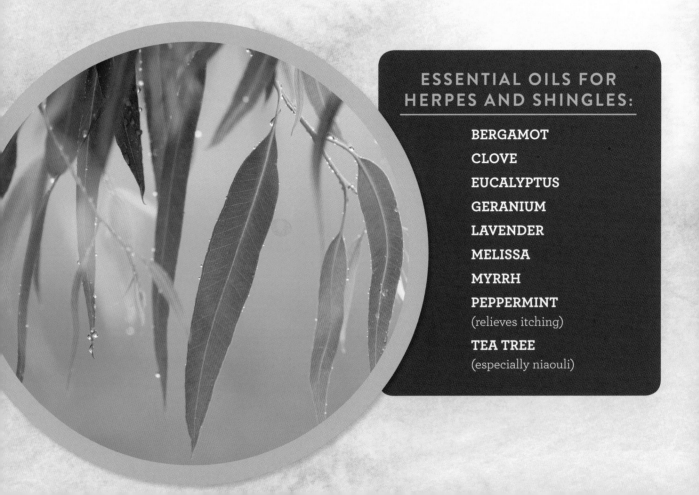

ESSENTIAL OILS FOR HERPES AND SHINGLES:

BERGAMOT

CLOVE

EUCALYPTUS

GERANIUM

LAVENDER

MELISSA

MYRRH

PEPPERMINT
(relieves itching)

TEA TREE
(especially niaouli)

HERPES RELIEF FORMULA 1

- 10 drops tea tree oil
- 5 drops myrrh oil
- 5 drops geranium or bergamot oil
- 2 drops peppermint oil (optional)
- 1/2 ounce carrier oil

Combine the ingredients and shake or stir well. Apply directly to affected area three to five times a day during an outbreak. The peppermint oil is optional because some people find it increases rather than dulls the pain. If you would prefer a less oily formula, you can substitute either rubbing alcohol or vodka for the carrier oil, but try a little first to make sure the alcohol doesn't sting too much.

Melissa oil is apparently a useful treatment for some herpes sufferers. The oil is applied neat, directly to the location of the outbreak. This remedy may be too irritating for the skin of some users, however. If you try this treatment, first dilute it with a carrier oil.

HERPES RELIEF FORMULA 2

- 8 drops tea tree oil
- 6 drops geranium oil
- 6 drops German chamomile oil
- 6 drops lavender oil
- 3 drops lemon oil

Combine ingredients and put one drop of mixture on a moist cotton ball. Dab gently over affected area.

HERPES RELIEF SITZ BATH

- 10 drops tea tree oil
- 10 drops lavender oil
- 6 drops melissa oil
- 5 drops geranium oil
- 2 tablespoons Epsom salts
- Enough warm water for sitz bath to cover problem areas

Combine ingredients in the water until mixed. Sit in bath as long as desired.

The essential oil of oregano is a powerful—and dangerous—substance. For that reason, we do not include it in the profile section. However, there is some anecdotal evidence, that application of the diluted oil may be an effective way to combat the herpes virus.

HIVES

Hives are rashlike, itchy skin bumps that are most often seen in children, but anyone can get them. They are often caused by a food allergy, although it may be difficult to diagnose at first because the reaction can occur hours or even a day after eating the culprit food. While it's a good idea to eliminate the allergen and build up the immune system, the immediate need is to stop the itching.

The essential oil of chamomile is an excellent first choice to treat hives, but if it's too expensive or you don't have any on hand, you can turn to an essential oil that decreases inflammation, such as lavender. The fragrance of either lavender or chamomile oil can also be very calming to someone who feels that they are going to go mad from the itching.

First wash off the skin with a warm aromatherapy wash. If the itching is not sufficiently relieved, apply the suggested paste (both recipes this page). A child who normally objects to having a poultice smeared on his or her skin will often accept this poultice because it so effectively stops the itching.

ESSENTIAL OILS FOR HIVES:

CHAMOMILE   **LAVENDER**   **PEPPERMINT**

HIVES SKIN WASH

- 5 drops chamomile or 10 drops lavender oil
- 2 drops peppermint oil
- 3 tablespoons baking soda
- 2 cups water (or use peppermint tea instead)

Combine the ingredients. If you are making a tea to use as the base instead of water, pour 2 1/2 cups of boiling water over 4 teaspoons of dried peppermint leaves, and steep 15 minutes. Strain out the herb. Add the remaining ingredients. Use a soft cloth or a skin sponge to apply on irritated skin until itching is alleviated. Chamomile is the best choice for this recipe, but it is expensive, so 10 drops of lavender essential oil can be substituted, if necessary.

HIVES PASTE

- 1/4 cup of the Hives Skin Wash
- 3 tablespoons bentonite clay

Stir the ingredients into a paste, and wait about five minutes for it to thicken. Apply to irritated skin with your fingers or a wooden tongue depressor. Let dry on skin, and leave for at least 45 minutes before washing off. Reapply for another 30 minutes if the area is still itching.

IMMUNE SYSTEM, WEAKENED

Many essential oils have a remarkable ability to both support the immune system and increase one's rate of healing. Some of these same essential oils are also powerful antiseptics. One way these oils fight infection is to stimulate the production of white corpuscles, which are part of the body's immune defense. Still other essential oils encourage new cell growth to promote faster healing. As an extra bonus, the regenerative properties of these essential oils improve the condition and tone of the skin. All can be used in conjunction with herbal remedies designed to improve immunity. Relaxation achieved through a massage or bath lowers stress, improves sleep, and thus stimulates the immune system.

One important way to assist your immune system is with a lymphatic massage that uses essential oils. Lymph nodes are located around the body, particularly in the throat, groin, breasts, and under the arms. They are like filtering centers for cleansing the blood. The lymphatic system moves cellular fluid through the system, cleansing the body of waste produced by the body's metabolic functions. Lemon, rosemary, and grapefruit are especially good at stimulating movement and supporting the cleansing action. A lymphatic massage involves deep strokes that work from the extremities toward the heart. You can even do this on yourself. Rub the oil up your arms to the lymph nodes in your armpits. From the center of your chest, rub again toward the armpit, and then down your neck. Massage your legs from your feet up to the groin.

ESSENTIAL OILS FOR THE IMMUNE SYSTEM:

BERGAMOT	LEMON	TEA TREE
CLOVE	MYRRH	THYME
GRAPEFRUIT	ROSEMARY	
LAVENDER	SAGE	

IMMUNITY BOOST MOUTH RINSE

- 1 drop clove oil
- 1 drop lemon oil
- 1 drop sage oil
- 1 drop tea tree oil
- 2 tablespoons cider vinegar
- Small glass of water, half full

Add ingredients to glass of water and gargle the entire contents, in batches. Do not swallow.

IMMUNE TONIC BLEND

- 6 drops lavender oil
- 6 drops bergamot oil
- 3 drops lemon oil
- 3 drops tea tree oil
- 2 drops myrrh oil
- 2 ounces carrier oil

Combine ingredients. Use as a general massage oil or over specific areas of the body that tend to develop physical problems. For example, if you come down with a lot of chest colds and flus, rub this blend over your chest. Use 1 to 2 teaspoons in a bath or 1 teaspoon in a foot bath. Without the carrier oil, this recipe is suitable for use in an aromatherapy diffuser, simmering pan of water, or potpourri cooker. Use in some form several times a day when trying to build up your own natural immunity.

LYMPH MASSAGE OIL

- 6 drops lemon oil
- 6 drops grapefruit oil
- 3 drops rosemary oil
- 2 drops bay laurel oil
- 2 ounces carrier oil

Combine ingredients. You can use this for any type of massage, but it is particularly effective when used in a lymphatic massage as described above. Remember that there are two essential oils named bay. This blend requires true bay laurel (*Laurus nobilis*), not the West Indian bay (*Pimenta racemosa*).

GERMS-BE-GONE ROOM SPRAY

- 8 drops cinnamon oil
- 8 drops clove oil
- 8 drops eucalyptus oil
- 8 drops lemon oil
- 8 drops rosemary oil
- 2 ounces witch hazel
- 8 ounces water

Fill spray bottle with all ingredients. Shake well before using.

IMMUNITY-BOOSTING DIFFUSION BLEND

- 3 drops clove oil
- 3 drops lemon oil
- 2 drops cinnamon oil
- 2 drops eucalyptus oil
- 1 drop rosemary oil
- Water

Fill diffuser with as much water as needed and add the oils. Turn diffuser on in a central location for maximum effect.

INDIGESTION/NAUSEA

Digestive woes such as belching, stomach pains, and intestinal gas are easily remedied with aromatherapy. A massage oil rubbed on the stomach is especially good for fussy children or anyone who refuses to swallow medicine.

Don't overlook the role that stress plays in impairing digestion. It can restrict the flow of digestive juices and constrict muscles in the digestive tract. No wonder so many people get a queasy stomach when encountering stressful situations. Tension is also thought to contribute to digestive complaints such as colitis and ulcers and most other digestive tract problems.

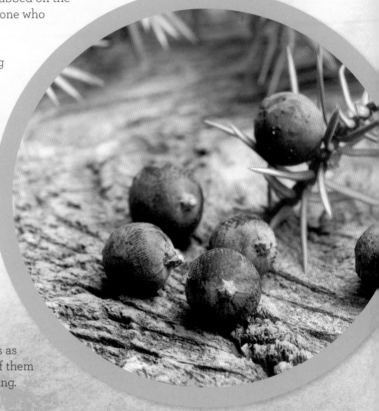

Aromatics start working at the first stage of digestion, when they signal the brain that food is coming. The response is almost immediate: Digestive juices are released in the mouth, stomach, and small intestine, preparing the way for proper assimilation. To aid digestion, add spices such as anise, basil, caraway, coriander, and fennel to your cooking, or drink a cup of peppermint, thyme, lemon balm, or chamomile tea. Even though many herb books describe these herbs as digestive stimulants, researchers found that most of them actually relax intestinal muscles and relieve cramping. This slower pace gives food more time to be adequately digested and, therefore, prevents gas. Thus, the same essential oils that improve poor appetite also relieve intestinal gas. These include peppermint, ginger, fennel, coriander, and dill.

Some oils have specialties: Rosemary improves poor food absorption and peppermint treats irritable bowel syndrome. Basil overcomes nausea from chemotherapy or radiation treatments (even when conventional drugs have little effect). Lemongrass is used in Brazil, the Caribbean, and much of South East Asia to relieve nervous digestion.

ESSENTIAL OILS FOR IMPROVED DIGESTION AND TO ELIMINATE GAS:

BLACK PEPPER	GINGER
CARAWAY	JUNIPER BERRY
CARDAMOM	LEMONGRASS
CHAMOMILE	PEPPERMINT
CLARY SAGE	ROSEMARY
CORIANDER	THYME
FENNEL	TURMERIC

TUMMY OIL 1

- 2 drops lemongrass oil
- 1 drop fennel oil
- 2 drops chamomile oil
- 2 ounces carrier oil

Combine the ingredients and massage over the abdominal area. This all-purpose formula will thwart indigestion, including nausea, gas, appetite loss, and motion sickness, as well as help improve appetite and digestion. You can also add 1 to 2 teaspoons to bathwater. Use as needed. Feel free to alter this formula by choosing other oils on the list, but be careful of hot oils like thyme, peppermint, and black pepper, especially in a bath since they can burn the skin.

TUMMY OIL 2

- 3 drops turmeric oil
- 2 drops basil oil
- 1 drop ginger oil
- 1 drop peppermint oil
- 2 ounces carrier oil

Combine the ingredients and follow the instructions for Tummy Oil 1.

QUICK NAUSEA FIX

It's utterly simple and surprisingly effective: fill a small glass halfway with lukewarm water and add two drops of peppermint oil. Stir and drink.

NAUSEA INHALATION REMEDY

- 20 drops bergamot oil
- 20 drops cardamom oil
- 20 drops grapefruit oil
- 15 drops spearmint oil
- 10 drops geranium oil
- 3 drops ginger oil

Combine all ingredients in a small glass bottle. When you're feeling nauseous, shake the bottle and take a few whiffs.

INSECT BITES

For mosquito or other insect bites that don't demand much attention, a simple dab of essential oil of lavender or tea tree provides relief from itching. Chamomile and lavender essential oils reduce swelling and inflammation, and diminish itching or other allergic response. Bentonite clay poultices are of great help for more painful stings or bites. As the clay dries, it pulls toxins to the skin's surface to keep them from spreading, and it pulls out pus or stingers embedded in the skin. Adding essential oil to clay keeps the clay reconstituted, preserved, and ready for an emergency. If an allergic reaction, such as excessive itching, swelling and inflammation, or difficulty breathing, occurs following a bite, call a doctor immediately.

ESSENTIAL OILS FOR BITES AND STINGS:

CHAMOMILE
LAVENDER
PEPPERMINT (stops itching)
TEA TREE

ESSENTIAL OILS THAT ARE INSECT REPELLENTS:

BIRCH
CEDARWOOD
CINNAMON
CLOVE
EUCALYPTUS
LAVENDER
LEMONGRASS (or citronella)
ORANGE
PATCHOULI
PEPPERMINT (repels ants)
PINE
SANDALWOOD

BUG-OFF REPELLENT

- 12 drops eucalyptus oil
- 12 drops lavender oil
- 6 drops cedarwood oil
- 6 drops geranium oil
- 6 drops lemongrass oil
- 6 drops rosewood oil
- 3 drops juniper oil
- 1 ounce rubbing alcohol or vodka

Mix ingredients together, and dab on exposed skin. This recipe contains a lot of essential oil and is highly concentrated, so don't use it like a massage oil. Rubbing alcohol is poisonous if drunk, so if you use it, be sure to mark the container accordingly. Pat on as needed. Since it won't harm fabrics (except silk), use some of it on your clothes so that you won't apply too much to your skin or absorb too much through the skin.

BITE AND STING POULTICE

- 12 drops lavender oil
- 5 drops chamomile oil
- 1 tablespoon bentonite clay
- 3 teaspoons distilled water

Put clay in the container to be stored. Add the water slowly, stirring more in as the clay absorbs it. Add essential oils, stirring to distribute them evenly. The resulting mixture should be a thick paste. If necessary, add more distilled water to achieve this consistency. Store the paste in a container with a tight lid to slow dehydration. It should last several months, but if the mixture starts to dry out, add a little distilled water to reconstitute it. Use as much and as often as needed.

INSOMNIA

Lack of sleep is a problem for millions of Americans. Feeling tired is only one of its difficulties. Sleep deprivation can eventually lead to chronic agitation, depression, dizziness, and headaches. Once you begin to get a good night's sleep, it's possible that most of these will clear up. For general soothing and relaxation, try jasmine or marjoram. For insomnia due to mental agitation or overwork, try clary sage or rose.

One of the most relaxing treatments for children—or anyone—before bed is a warm lavender and chamomile essential oil bath. For complete relaxation, follow the bath with an aromatherapy massage. Even a simple back or foot rub often does the trick.

You can also send children off to dreamland with a "dilly pillow." This is a small herb-filled pillow of lavender, hops, melissa, chamomile, and dill. European children used to regularly sleep with these pillows, while adults often slept on pillows stuffed simply with dried hops. Unlike most herbs, hops actually get better with age (up to a point), since exposure to air increases the sedative effects. So you don't have to worry about diminishing potency if you keep them in a pillowcase. That said, dried hops may begin to give off a "stinky feet" aroma with age and oxidization. This is mainly due to the valerianic acid (the same substance found in the notoriously stinky valerian).

ESSENTIAL OILS FOR INSOMNIA:

BERGAMOT	HOPS	ROSE
CHAMOMILE	JASMINE	SANDALWOOD
CLARY SAGE	LAVENDER	YLANG YLANG
FRANKINCENSE	MARJORAM	

In lieu of a hops pillow, you can add 3 or 4 drops of hops essential oil to a tissue and place it next to your head when you go to bed. You may also diffuse it at bedtime or add a few drops to your bath. Studies have shown that the combination of hops and valerian is a particularly efficacious remedy.

ZZZZ FORMULA 1

- 15 drops bergamot oil
- 10 drops lavender oil
- 10 drops sandalwood oil
- 3 drops frankincense
- 2 drops ylang ylang oil
- 4 ounces carrier oil

Combine the ingredients and use as a massage oil, or put 2 teaspoons in your bath. Feeling extravagant? Then add 2 drops of your choice of an expensive essential oil such as jasmine or rose. Without the carrier oil, this recipe is suitable for use in an aromatherapy diffuser, simmering pan of water, or potpourri cooker. Treat yourself every night before bed as a surefire way to drift sweetly off to the Land of Nod.

ZZZZ FORMULA 2

- 15 drops Roman chamomile
- 10 drops lavender oil
- 10 drops frankincense oil
- 5 drops marjoram oil
- 5 drops hops oil
- 4 ounces carrier oil

Combine ingredients and follow the instructions for ZZZZ Formula 1.

HOPS SLEEP PILLOW

- 1/4 cup hops
- 1/8 cup chamomile flowers
- 1/8 cup lavender flowers (optional)
- 1/8 cup dill weed (optional)
- 2 pieces of suitable cloth material about eight inches square

Sew material together around the edge, leaving enough room to insert a tablespoon. Fold over so stitching is inside. Combine the dried herbs and spoon them into the pillow. Sew up the opening. Lay the hops pillow under your regular sleeping pillow. If you are feeling creative, you can make the pillow any shape or size. Just make more of this recipe to fill it. A drop or two of the essential oils of hops, lavender, chamomile, or dill can be added periodically to the fabric to refresh the scent.

SLEEP AID DIFFUSER BLEND

- 4 drops marjoram oil
- 3 drops cedarwood oil
- 3 drops lavender oil
- 1 drop vetiver oil

Fill diffuser with water, add all oils, and run diffuser just prior to bedtime.

JOINT PAIN

A liniment heats the skin and underlying muscles and joints to relieve pain. The base of a liniment may be either rubbing alcohol or an edible alcohol such as vodka. If you do use rubbing alcohol, remember that it is toxic to drink, so label it accordingly. Alcohol is cooling and quickly evaporates, leaving no oily residue. Occasionally, though, a person will prefer using a carrier oil base, making the liniment more like a concentrated massage oil. Oil heats up faster and will stay on the skin longer, making it better for massages.

Essential oils such as cinnamon, peppermint, and clove give a liniment its heating action. All skin-heating preparations, including Tiger Balm and White Flower Oil, contain peppermint and/or camphor, which stimulate both hot and cold reactions in nerve endings in the skin. The brain registers these sensations at the same time. The contrast between the two messages makes a liniment seem much hotter than it really is.

The most effective liniments also contain muscle-relaxing and inflammation-reducing essential oils such as rosemary, marjoram, and lavender. They penetrate into the skin to work directly on the muscle.

For arthritis, rheumatism, and other inflammatory conditions, use chamomile, marjoram, birch, and ginger in a massage oil. These same oils can also be added to a pain-relieving bath. For arthritic hands or feet, try a daily hand or foot bath.

ESSENTIAL OILS FOR JOINT PAIN:

BIRCH	JUNIPER BERRY
CHAMOMILE	MARJORAM
CLOVE	MYRRH
CYPRESS	PEPPERMINT
FIR	ROSEMARY
GINGER	

ESSENTIAL OILS FOR HEATING LINIMENTS:

CINNAMON

CLOVE

EUCALYPTUS

PEPPERMINT

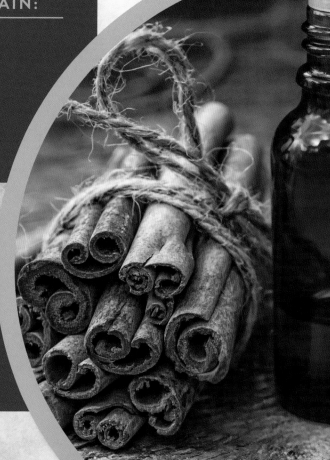

JOINT PAIN LINIMENT

- 8 drops eucalyptus oil
- 8 drops peppermint oil
- 8 drops rosemary oil
- 4 drops cinnamon leaf oil
- 4 drops juniper berry oil
- 4 drops marjoram oil
- 2 ounces alcohol (either rubbing or vodka)

Mix ingredients. Shake or stir a few times daily for three days to disperse the essential oils in the alcohol. This formula is stronger than a typical massage oil, so don't use it over a large area of the body. Instead, concentrate on painful joints. It will also work well as a warm-up liniment before exercising or heavy physical work to help prevent muscles from cramping or becoming stiff. If preferred, the alcohol in this recipe can be replaced with a carrier oil. Use several times a day as needed.

ARTHRITIS RUB OIL

- 2 drops birch oil
- 2 drops cypress oil
- 2 drops eucalyptus oil
- 2 drops frankincense oil
- 2 drops peppermint oil
- 2 tablespoons carrier oil

Combine all ingredients. Massage mixture into problem areas.

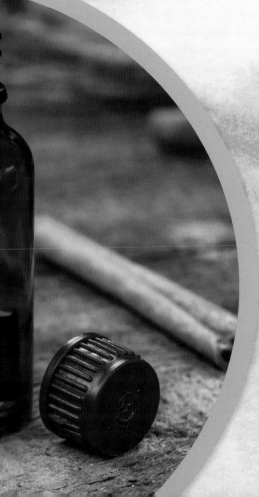

RHEUMATIC EASE RUB OIL

- 3 drops turmeric oil
- 3 drops myrrh oil
- 2 drops frankincense oil
- 2 drops ginger oil
- 2 drops orange oil
- 1 drop peppermint oil
- 2 tablespoons carrier oil

Combine all ingredients. Massage mixture into problem areas.

JOINT INFLAMMATION AND STRAIN RUB OIL

- 3 drops Roman chamomile oil
- 2 drops helichrysum oil
- 2 drops lavender oil
- 2 drops marjoram oil
- 2 drops turmeric oil
- 1 drop rosemary oil
- 2 tablespoons carrier oil

Combine all ingredients. Massage mixture into problem areas.

MEMORY

Researchers have learned that memory recall at least doubles when a past event is associated with a smell. That's why a whiff of a fragrance can send you back in time and carry with it images and feelings associated with that event. Next time you need help accessing some elusive fact, aromatherapy can trigger your memory. Rosemary, for instance, has a long history of increasing memory, concentration, and even creativity.

And modern Japanese research confirms rosemary is a brain stimulant. Other mental stimulants are sage, basil, and bay laurel.

Inhale one of the recommended essential oils while you are studying for a test or attending a class. Then, when you need to recall the information, simply smell the same scent.

ESSENTIAL OILS FOR MEMORY:

ROSEMARY	CLARY SAGE

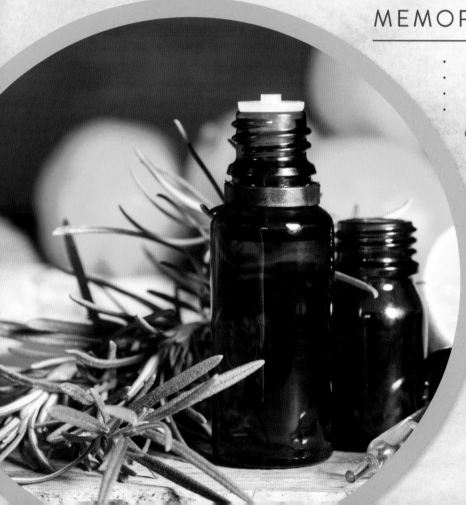

MEMORY FORMULA

- 10 drops rosemary oil
- 6 drops lemon oil
- 1 drop clary sage oil
- 2 ounces distilled water

Combine ingredients, and use as a spray. Without water, this formula can be used in an aromatherapy diffuser or dabbed on a tissue to smell while you are studying. The lemon oil provides both alertness and a pleasing scent.

MENOPAUSE

Not all women experience problems at menopause. But those who do will find aromatherapy at least part of the answer to them. Ideally it will be used in combination with a complete herbal program. Menopause symptoms include hot flashes, bone fragility, confusion, depression, and a dry, less elastic vagina with a thinner lining—all thought to be caused by the erratic activity or insufficiency of hormones. Several essential oils that contain hormone-like substances related to estrogen are helpful during menopause. These include clary sage, anise, fennel, cypress, angelica, coriander, sage, and to a lesser degree, basil. Such essential oils, along with peppermint and lemon, will help relieve hot flashes. Since essential oils go right through the skin, applying them to fatty areas of the body where hormones are manufactured and stored will create the most direct effect. Of course, any massage is itself very therapeutic. A bath is also a wonderful way to receive the benefits of these oils.

Geranium, neroli, and lavender are balance hormones and also help modify menopausal symptoms. They are traditionally used in European face creams to reduce aging and wrinkles. As a rejuvenation cream, these oils not only perk up a dry complexion, they make a good cream to counter vaginal dryness. Add some vitamin E oil, which improves the strength and flexibility of the vaginal lining while quickly healing abrasions that can occur during intercourse when the lining is too dry. In addition to aromatherapy, try dietary and herbal treatments to alleviate some of menopause's unpleasant symptoms.

ESSENTIAL OILS THAT AFFECT ESTROGEN AND BALANCE HORMONES:

| CYPRESS | LAVENDER | ROSE |
| GERANIUM | NEROLI | CLARY SAGE |

ESSENTIAL OILS THAT EASE HOT FLASHES:

| CLARY SAGE | LEMON | PEPPERMINT |

ESSENTIAL OILS FOR EMOTIONAL UPS AND DOWNS:

| CHAMOMILE | JASMINE | NEROLI |

MENOPAUSE BODY OIL

- 6 drops lemon oil
- 5 drops geranium oil
- 2 drops clary sage oil
- 1 drop angelica oil
- 1 drop jasmine oil
- 2 ounces carrier oil or body lotion

Combine the ingredients. Use at least once a day as a massage oil, in a lotion, or in a bath (add 2 teaspoons to the bathwater). If this formula is too oily for you, add the same essential oils to 2 ounces of a commercial body lotion instead. The best type to use is an unscented, basic lotion that contains ingredients that are as natural as possible.

REJUVENATION OIL

- 6 drops geranium oil
- 6 drops lavender
- 1 drop neroli
- 1500 units vitamin E oil
- 1 ounce carrier oil

Combine ingredients. For the vitamin E, either buy the liquid vitamin or open vitamin capsules and empty the contents into your preparation. Apply to both the inside and outside of the vagina as needed. You can also stir these essential oils into a prepared cream.

QUICK RESET FORMULA

- 20 drops clary sage oil
- 20 drops ylang ylang oil
- 10 drops basil oil
- 10 drops Roman chamomile
- 10 drops thyme oil
- 5 drops geranium oil
- 1 ounce carrier oil

Combine all ingredients. When needed, shake bottle thoroughly and apply to the neck.

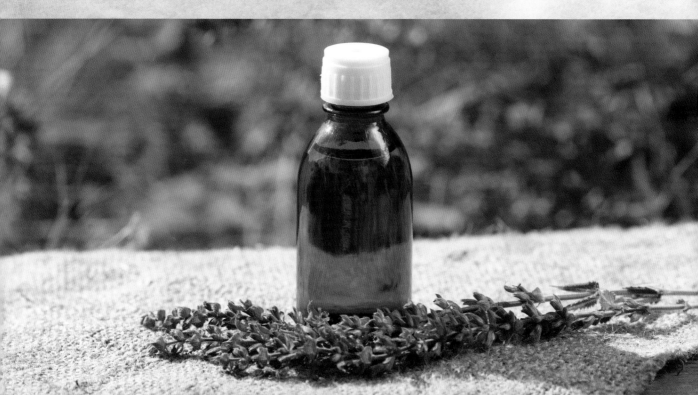

MUSCLE CRAMPS

Muscles can hurt after a vigorous day of exercise or work, especially if you aren't exercising on a regular basis and then really go for it. Activities that you repeat daily can also tighten muscles and cause them to cramp. The Cramp Relief Oil formula (page 226) is excellent for lower back or shoulder pain, tight muscles from working at a computer, or the aftereffects of physical exercise. Even menstrual cramps, which are really little more than the cramping of the uterine muscle, respond well to this remedy. By the way, this same recipe can be used as a first-aid treatment along with ice on sprains and bruises. The sooner it is applied, the better. It reduces the swelling and pain and promotes faster healing.

Recent medical thinking tends to support using a liniment containing heating oils to increase blood circulation and warmth to an area before exercising rather than waiting until afterward. By doing so, the liniment works like a mini warm-up for the muscles. You'll still want to do your warm-up exercises, but the combination will give you extra warmth, helping to prevent muscle cramps. Then, if your muscles do cramp, use the cramp relief oil below to relax them.

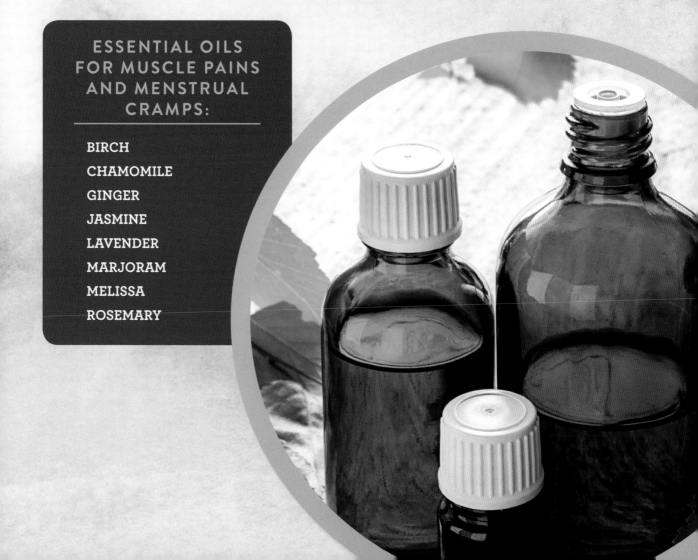

ESSENTIAL OILS FOR MUSCLE PAINS AND MENSTRUAL CRAMPS:

BIRCH

CHAMOMILE

GINGER

JASMINE

LAVENDER

MARJORAM

MELISSA

ROSEMARY

CRAMP RELIEF OIL

- 12 drops lavender oil
- 6 drops marjoram oil
- 4 drops Roman chamomile oil
- 4 drops ginger oil
- 2 ounces carrier oil

Combine ingredients. Apply throughout the day as often as needed over the cramping area. This formula is also excellent for the lower back pain that sometimes accompanies menstrual cramps. It works well when made with any carrier oil, but if you can, use St. John's wort oil instead, as it is excellent for sore muscles. You can buy a ready-made version online and it can often be found at health food stores.

REJUVENESCENT MUSCLE OIL

- 10 drops helichrysum oil
- 7 drops frankincense oil
- 4 drops cajuput oil
- 4 drops juniper oil
- 3 drops rosemary oil
- 2 ounces carrier oil

Combine ingredients. Massage into sore spots at least twice a day.

BACK AND SHOULDER RUB

- 9 drops rosemary oil
- 8 drops spruce oil
- 6 drops Roman chamomile oil
- 4 drops birch oil
- 2 drops peppermint oil
- 2 ounces carrier oil

Combine ingredients. Massage into back and shoulders.

PULLED MUSCLE PAIN RELIEF BLEND

- 9 drops German chamomile oil
- 6 drops frankincense oil
- 6 drops marjoram oil
- 4 drops ginger oil
- 4 drops clove oil
- 2 ounces carrier oil

NAUSEA/MOTION SICKNESS

That queasy feeling in the stomach that signals nausea can be caused by quite a few different problems. Topping the list are motion sickness, food poisoning, the flu, headaches, emotional upset, anxiety, medications, and pregnancy. Peppermint and ginger ease both nausea and motion sickness. Chamomile and fennel relax the stomach and soothe burning irritation and inflammation. Basil overcomes nausea from chemotherapy or radiation treatments (even when conventional drugs have little effect). Lemongrass is used in Brazil, the Caribbean, and much of South East Asia to relieve nervous digestion. Sometimes the smell alone of such essential oils as peppermint, ginger, or basil is enough to quell nausea. If not, use them in a massage oil where they will enter the bloodstream.

Prefer the taste of peppermint? It's usually at the top of the list for preventing motion sickness and works equally well for general stomach upsets. While essential oils are usually too potent to ingest, two drops of peppermint oil in a glass of water is a time-honored remedy. If you are prone to motion sickness, consider carrying a small vial of peppermint oil with you on your next airplane flight, boat ride, or any form of travel. Or try mixing peppermint with some of the other oils (in very small quantities, of course) mentioned below.

ESSENTIAL OILS FOR NAUSEA AND MOTION SICKNESS:

CORIANDER

GINGER

PEPPERMINT

SANDALWOOD

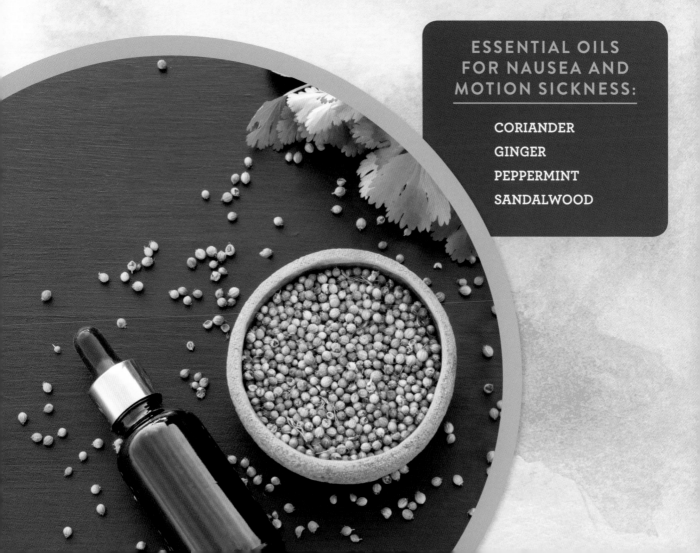

NERVE PAIN

The nerves in your body register pain, so when nerves are damaged, the condition will be quite painful. Injured nerves take a long time to regenerate, but aromatherapy treatments can help with the process. They initially relieve pain, and people who use them appear to heal more quickly than others.

Essential oils of lavender, chamomile, and marjoram are excellent at easing the pain of a pinched nerve or sciatica. The lesser-known essential oil helichrysum (the *italicum* variety) is specific for this condition. Apply the oil directly on the back or hip to reduce pain. It is also wonderful on painful shingles. People with serious nerve-related problems, such as multiple sclerosis and chronic fatigue syndrome, get noticeable pain relief from the Nerve Pain Oil recipe featured here. For carpal tunnel syndrome, rub this oil into the wrists. Since nerve conditions can be difficult to heal, talk to someone skilled in natural medicine for more ideas on how to treat them.

ESSENTIAL OILS FOR NERVE PAIN:

CHAMOMILE	PEPPERMINT
LAVENDER	SANDALWOOD
MARJORAM	

NERVE PAIN OIL

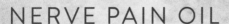

- 4 drops chamomile oil
- 3 drops marjoram oil
- 3 drops helichrysum oil
- 2 drops lavender oil
- 1 ounce carrier oil or St. John's wort oil

Combine the ingredients. Apply as needed throughout the day for pain relief. This formula is even more effective if St. John's wort oil is used.

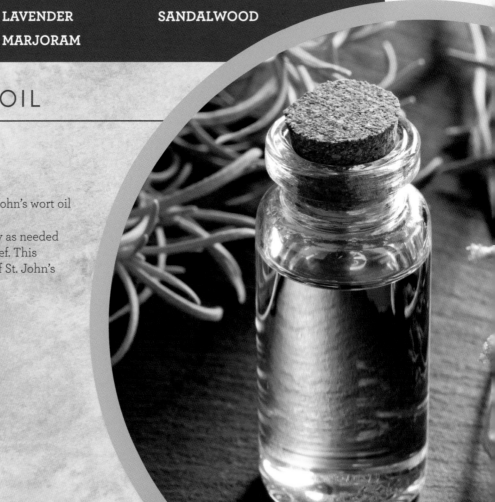

POISON OAK/IVY/SUMAC

The infamous, extremely itchy rash that is caused by exposure to urushiol, the chemical culprit in poison oak, poison ivy, and poison sumac, is a type of dermatitis that calls for special aromatherapy care. Make sure to use a vinegar base, as oil-based products aren't usually recommended in the first stages of the outbreak. However, some people find that a lotion relieves the later dry stage.

Choose essential oils that slow the inflammation and ease the itching. Peppermint may seem an unlikely essential oil to use, but the menthol it contains actually relieves the painful burning and itching that accompany the rash.

If you can, first soak the affected area in a tepid oatmeal bath. Then apply the remedy we offer here.

OAT BATH

- 3 drops of any of these oils: chamomile, cypress, geranium, lavender
- 1 drop peppermint oil
- 4 cups quick-cooking oats (they dissolve best)
- 1 cup Epsom salts
- a square of muslin or double-layered cheesecloth

Add the essential oils to the oats and put them into the cloth, which should be tied to form a bag. Put all ingredients in a lukewarm bath and soak yourself in it. Do this several times a day if it helps. Or mix a smaller amount of oats dissolved in hot water with the essential oils, and sponge it on.

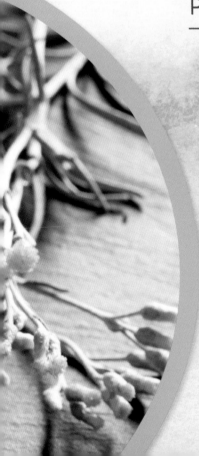

POISON OAK/IVY/SUMAC REMEDY

- 3 drops lavender oil
- 3 drops cypress oil
- 3 drops peppermint oil
- 1/2 teaspoon salt
- 1 tablespoon warm water
- 1 tablespoon apple cider vinegar

Dissolve the salt in the water and vinegar; then add the other ingredients. Shake well to disperse and again before each use. Apply externally as needed to the rash.

PREMENSTRUAL SYNDROME (PMS)

Premenstrual syndrome, better known as PMS, is a collection of many different symptoms that typically begin several days or even a week before menstruation. The host of symptoms includes water retention, breast swelling and tenderness, depression, irritability, mood swings, and headaches. Not all women who get PMS experience all of these symptoms, but any one of them can greatly alter one's life while going through it.

In many ways, aromatherapy is ideal to treat PMS. Taking time out to lounge in an aromatic bath or getting a massage with a fragrant oil helps most women tremendously. For depression and mood swings associated with PMS, nothing can beat clary sage.

The essential oils of neroli, rose, and jasmine may be expensive, but their heavenly fragrances help dispel moodiness and irritability.

For the excessive bloating and swollen breasts of PMS, use the essential oils of juniper berry, patchouli, grapefruit, and carrot seed. Another good oil for this is birch, which is also a natural pain reliever. Use juniper berry if you experience water retention. If headache is among your PMS symptoms, try an inhalation of lavender or marjoram. For best results with any PMS or menstruation remedy, begin using it a couple of days before you experience any symptoms. Refer also to the sections on fatigue, acne, and menstrual cramps.

ESSENTIAL OILS FOR PMS:

CHAMOMILE	MARJORAM
CLARY SAGE	NEROLI
GERANIUM	ROSE
JASMINE	

ESSENTIAL OILS FOR BLOATING:

BIRCH	LAVENDER
JUNIPER BERRY	PATCHOULI

MOOD OIL

- 9 drops geranium oil
- 6 drops chamomile oil
- 3 drops clary sage oil
- 3 drops angelica oil
- 2 drops marjoram oil
- 2 ounces carrier oil

Combine the ingredients. Use daily as a massage oil or add 1 to 2 teaspoons to a bath. This recipe improves your mood even if you don't have PMS. To make it more elegant and effective, add 1 or 2 drops of neroli, rose, or jasmine. Without the carrier oil, you can use this in a diffuser or simply carry around a vial of it to smell as needed.

BLOATING AND HEADACHE RELIEF OIL

- 6 drops lavender oil
- 3 drops juniper berry oil
- 2 drops birch oil
- 1 drop patchouli oil (optional)

Combine ingredients. Use as a massage oil or add 1 to 2 teaspoons to your bath or 1 teaspoon to a foot bath. Don't use the patchouli if you don't like the smell; it can easily overwhelm a formula.

BALANCE BATH BLEND

- 3 drops clary sage oil
- 2 drops chamomile oil
- 2 drops geranium oil
- 2 drops lavender oil
- 1 cup Epsom salts

Mix all ingredients together first, then add to your warm bath.

DIFFUSE AND DEFUSE BLEND

- 5 drops orange oil
- 3 drops frankincense oil
- 1 drop ylang ylang oil

Add ingredients to your diffuser and use at times of stress and irritability.

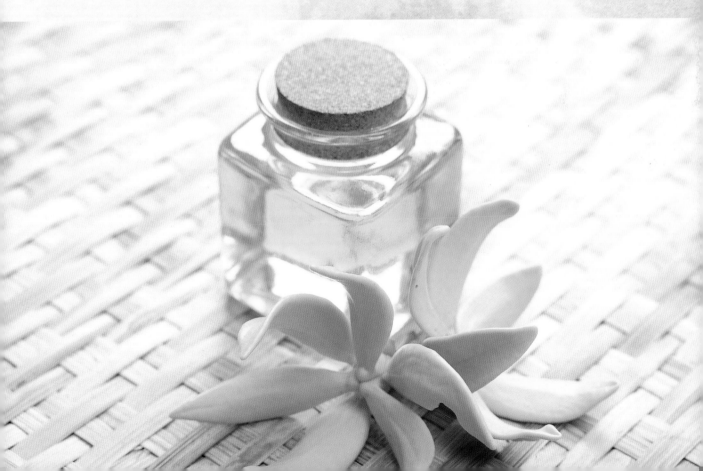

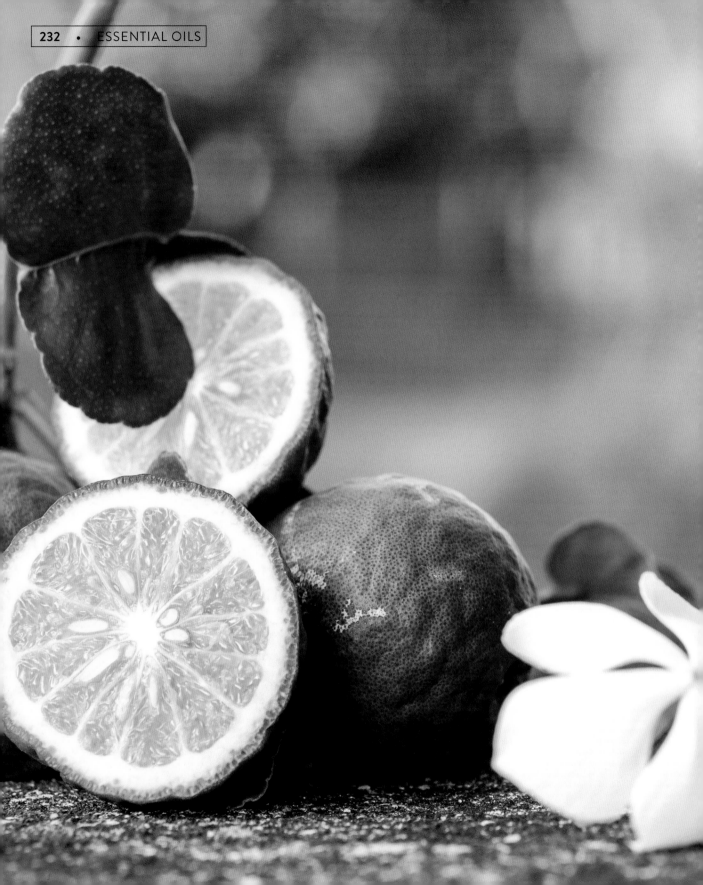

SORE THROAT/LARYNGITIS

A bacterial infection or lots of singing, talking, or yelling can cause a sore throat. At times, the throat can be so inflamed and painful that it becomes difficult to swallow or talk. If the inflammation is in the voice box, you can easily come down with laryngitis, in which your voice is reduced to a hoarse whisper or it even may become impossible to talk at all.

For centuries, European singers have known the secret to preserving their voices with aromatherapy and herbal remedies. Their most popular sore throat and laryngitis cure has been to gargle with a marjoram herb tea that has been sweetened with honey. You can use the essential oil of marjoram to make a similar remedy. As both an antiseptic and anti-inflammatory, marjoram is a good choice. Other essential oils or herb teas to use as a gargle are sage, hyssop, and thyme, all of which kill bacterial infections.

Any of these essential oils can easily be gargled or sprayed into the throat. This brings the antibacterial and soothing essential oils into direct contact with the bacteria responsible for causing a sore throat or laryngitis. In an emergency, a few drops of essential oil diluted in two ounces of water may also be used.

Both lavender and eucalyptus work so well in an aromatherapy steam to recover your voice that you must remind yourself to not overstress it until your throat fully recovers. And don't forget the old standard of a hot drink made with fresh lemon juice and honey.

ESSENTIAL OILS FOR SORE THROAT:

BERGAMOT	LEMON	SANDALWOOD
EUCALYPTUS	MARJORAM	TEA TREE
LAVENDER	SAGE	THYME

THROAT SPRAY OR GARGLE

- 4 drops marjoram oil
- 1/2 cup warm water
- 1/2 teaspoon salt

Combine ingredients. Shake well to dissolve the salt and disperse the oils before spraying or gargling. Gargle every half hour at first and then several times a day.

NECK WRAP

- 2 drops bergamot oil
- 2 drops lavender oil
- 1 drop tea tree oil
- 2 cups hot water

Mix the water with the essential oils. While still warm, soak a soft cloth, preferably flannel, in the water and wring it out. Wrap it around the neck. Cover with a towel (thin enough to be comfortable) to hold in the heat. Remove before it becomes cold. Use throughout the day as often as you wish.

STRESS

Stress is part of life. It has a powerful effect on the body and takes its toll on both mental and physical well-being. It can cause headaches, nervous indigestion, or heart palpitations. Medical research now says that stress may be largely responsible for causing or at least promoting more serious disorders such as heart disease and allergies. Stress also overworks the adrenal glands. Repeated release of an overabundance of adrenaline from these glands eventually disrupts the delicate balance of your brain chemistry and hormonal production. Initially this will make you feel like you are always on edge. Eventually, the adrenal glands become exhausted and the opposite reaction occurs. You become tired, sluggish, listless, and emotions may easily fly out of control.

It is not always easy to avoid stress, but there are ways you can cope with it better. Fortunately, aromatherapy offers some of the best types of natural prescriptions for easing stress. For starters, incorporate these scents into your life in as many ways as possible, especially by using the ideas and recipes given throughout this book.

When applying the oil formulas, give yourself several minutes of slow, deep, even breathing while you imagine how, with each breath, the oil molecules are entering your bloodstream, and spreading throughout your body, relaxing tight muscles and alleviating tensions and strain. These moments will soon become one of your favorite times of the day.

Lavender, bergamot, marjoram, sandalwood, lemon, and chamomile were found (in that order) to relax brain waves. Doctors Giovanni Gatti and Renato Cayola discovered that the most sedating oils for their patients were neroli, petitgrain, chamomile, valerian, and opopanax (which is similar to myrrh). Aromatherapists find ylang ylang another potent relaxant.

ESSENTIAL OILS THAT RELAX AND SEDATE:

BERGAMOT	LEMON	ORANGE
CHAMOMILE	MARJORAM	SANDALWOOD
LAVENDER	NEROLI	YLANG YLANG

RELAXING BATH

- 2 drops bergamot oil
- 1 drop petitgrain oil

Add oils directly to the bath and stir to distribute.

RELAXING MASSAGE OIL

- 10 drops lavender oil
- 6 drops chamomile oil
- 4 drops ylang ylang oil
- 4 drops sandalwood oil
- 2 ounces carrier oil

Combine ingredients. Use as a massage oil as needed, or add 1 or 2 teaspoons to your bath or 1 teaspoon to a footbath. To add sophistication and an extra lift to this blend, add 1 drop of neroli essential oil. For children less than 8 years of age, use half the quantity of essential oil recommended. Without the carrier oil, this combination can be used in an aromatherapy diffuser, simmering pan of water, or a potpourri cooker, or you can add it to 2 ounces of water for an air spray. Use daily and as often as you like.

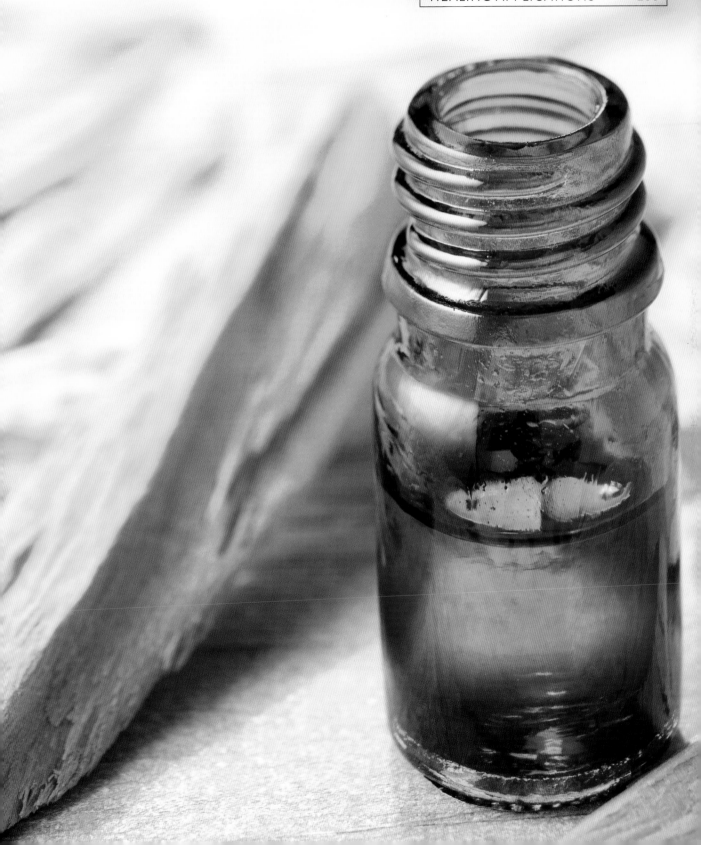

TENDINITIS

Tendons are the thick tissues that bind bone and muscle. Although extremely strong, they can be damaged. Inflammation and micro-tearing occur with overuse and overextension. Tendinitis—stiffness, pain, and swelling—is the result. Rest, hot and cold therapy, and essential oils are often enough to alleviate the symptoms and allow the body to heal itself. However, you should always seek professional treatment if the pain or swelling is severe, or if your range of motion is reduced. Ruptured tendons may require surgery.

ESSENTIAL OILS THAT EASE TENDINITIS:

BIRCH	FRANKINCENSE	LAVENDER
CHAMOMILE	HELICHRYSUM	MARJORAM
EUCALYPTUS	JUNIPER	PEPPERMINT

COOLING RUB

- 4 drops eucalyptus oil
- 4 drops peppermint oil
- 1 teaspoon carrier oils

Combine ingredients. Rub mixture into affected area. Repeat every 3 hours as necessary.

DEEP TISSUE REPAIR RUB

- 20 drops helichrysum oil
- 10 drops frankincense oil
- 10 drops German chamomile oil
- 5 drops juniper oil
- 5 drops lavender oil
- 5 drops peppermint oil
- 1 ounce carrier oil

Combine ingredients. Rub mixture into affected area. Repeat every 3 hours as necessary.

TOOTHACHE

For more than a century, clove oil has been used to ease all types of tooth pain, at least until you can get to the dentist. Even dentists themselves still recommend clove oil to their patients, and it is found in several dental preparations. In an emergency, simply put a clove bud in your mouth where it hurts the most. As it softens, mash the clove gently with your teeth to release the oil, and suck on it.

To relieve teething pain, rub the child's gums with a little Toothache Oil on your finger. Clove oil can be hot, so try it in your own mouth first. If it is still too hot, dilute it with more olive oil before putting it in your baby's mouth.

ESSENTIAL OILS FOR TOOTHACHE:

CHAMOMILE   CLOVE

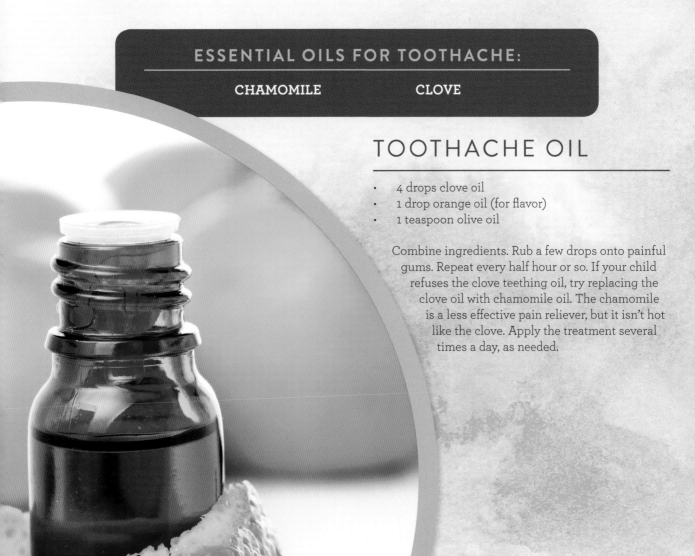

TOOTHACHE OIL

- 4 drops clove oil
- 1 drop orange oil (for flavor)
- 1 teaspoon olive oil

Combine ingredients. Rub a few drops onto painful gums. Repeat every half hour or so. If your child refuses the clove teething oil, try replacing the clove oil with chamomile oil. The chamomile is a less effective pain reliever, but it isn't hot like the clove. Apply the treatment several times a day, as needed.

UTERINE PROBLEMS

There are a variety of uterine problems, including endometriosis, pelvic inflammatory disease, cervical dysplasia, and serious menstrual cramps, for which aromatherapy is useful as an adjunct to other treatments. Endometriosis is a displacement of the uterine lining on the outside of the uterus or other areas where it doesn't belong. This condition causes inflammation and scarring and can be very painful. Pelvic inflammatory disease, nicknamed PID, is a very serious problem because it is usually a result of a difficult-to-treat infection in the uterine tissue. Cervical dysplasia is precancerous cell growth on the cervix. Menstrual cramps are muscle cramping that occurs in the uterus during menstruation; for some women, the cramps are so painful that they are debilitating.

A massage oil made from relaxing essential oils like lavender and chamomile helps relieve the inflammation, discomfort, and even the pain of most uterine problems. Rosemary promotes circulation. Two treatments handy for encouraging uterine healing are the castor oil pack and the sitz bath combined with aromatherapy. No one can explain exactly how these treatments work, but herbalists and aromatherapists have seen what a difference they can make. The sitz bath requires two tubs large enough to sit in so that water covers the abdomen. It is best if these can both fit into your bathtub, where spilling water won't be a problem. Fill one with hot water and the other with cold. You can also use the bathtub for hot water and have a plastic tub next to it on the floor for cold. Switch back and forth between the hot and cold about four times. Four minutes in the hot and one minute in the cold is tolerable and actually feels good after a few rounds. You will soon want the hot hotter and the cold colder!

A recent study from Washington University found that a castor oil pack improves the action of the immune system in the pelvic area when placed on the abdomen.

ESSENTIAL OILS FOR UTERINE PROBLEMS:

CHAMOMILE   **LAVENDER**   **ROSEMARY**

SITZ BATH

- 5 drops rosemary oil
- 5 drops lavender oil

Add the essential oils to the hot bath only. Sit in a tub with the hot water up to your waist for five to ten minutes. Then switch to a tub of cold water for at least one minute. The large plastic tubs sold at hardware stores work well for this. Continue for two to five rounds. Do this treatment every day, if possible, or at least twice a week.

CASTOR OIL PACK

- 8 drops lavender oil
- 1/4 cup castor oil
- soft cloth

Combine lavender and castor oils. Soak the cloth in oil. Fold the cloth, and place it in a baking dish in the oven set at 350°F for about 15 minutes. It should be quite warm, but not uncomfortable. Place the folded cloth directly over the uterus and cover with a towel to keep it warm. (Placing a hot water bottle or heating pad on top and surrounding it all with a towel works even better.) Afterward, rinse off the oil. Keep the pack on for 30 to 60 minutes, two or three times per week until the condition has cleared.

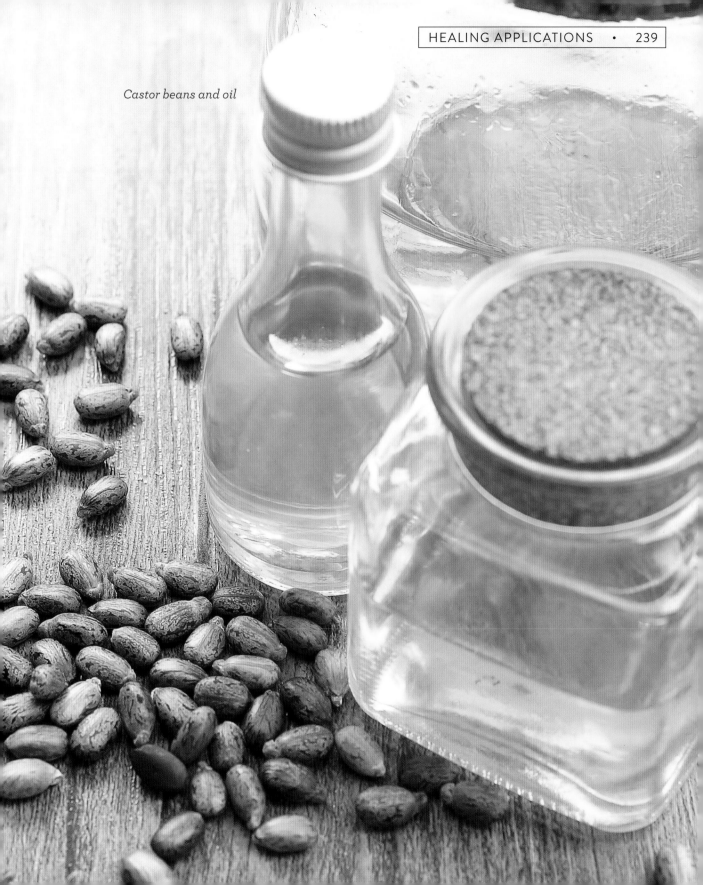

Castor beans and oil

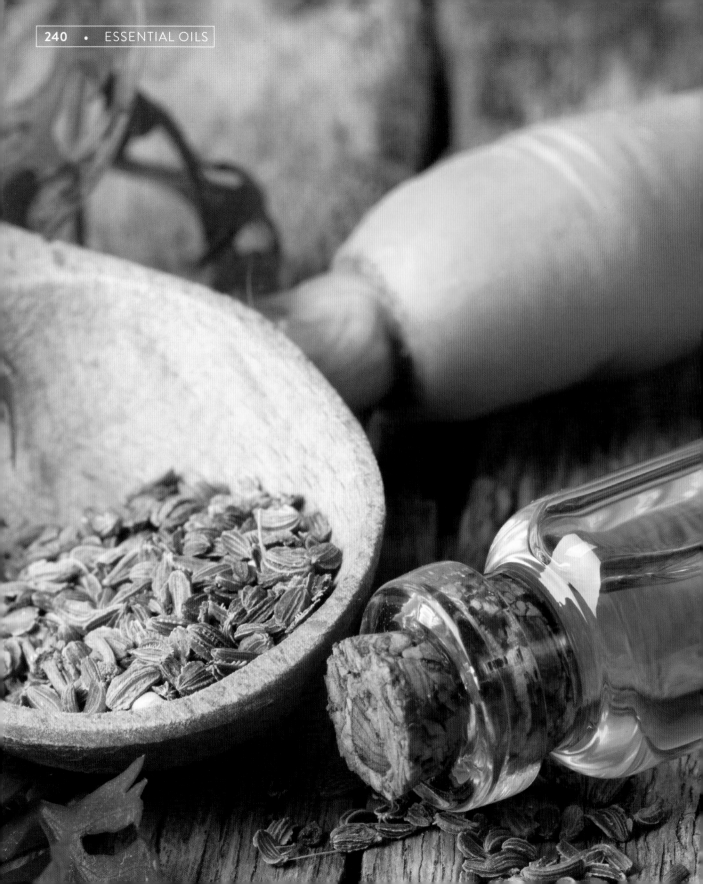

VARICOSE VEINS/ HEMORRHOIDS

Varicose veins and hemorrhoids both occur when circulating blood slows down on its way back to the heart. Blood relies on muscles in your legs and pelvis to push it back to the heart—not an easy task if you spend your day sitting or standing for long periods. If you are very overweight, pregnant, or constipated, or if you wear skin-tight pants or a girdle, blood flow through your pelvic area is also restricted. Over time, this extra blood load causes veins to weaken and stretch, resulting in extended veins on the legs that show as blue streaks running up and down the leg or as hemorrhoids, which are dilated and protruding veins in or around the anus.

There is usually little treatment outside of surgery that doctors can offer anyone who has varicose veins or hemorrhoids. However, essential oils of chamomile, palmarosa, myrtle, frankincense, and cypress reduce enlarged veins, ease the inflammation, and lessen pain. Massage oils containing these essential oils can be gently rubbed on the veins. When massaging the legs, use upward strokes that go with the blood flow, and be sure you don't push too deeply since these veins are already fragile.

If varicose veins and hemorrhoids reach the point at which the skin breaks and ulcers form, try applying a compress of lavender essential oil. Carrot seed essential oil specifically helps conditions where there is inflammation associated with enlarged veins.

ESSENTIAL OILS FOR VARICOSE VEINS:

CHAMOMILE	FRANKINCENSE	LAVENDER
CYPRESS	JUNIPER BERRY	MYRRH

LAVENDER CARROT COMPRESS

- 3 drops carrot seed oil
- 3 drops chamomile oil
- 3 drops lavender oil
- 1 cup cold water
- 1 teaspoon St. John's wort oil

Combine ingredients. Stir a soft cloth in the solution, wring it out, and place it over itching or broken varicose veins or hemorrhoids as often as practical. It can be used daily.

VEIN OIL

- 10 drops palmarosa oil
- 8 drops cypress oil
- 7 drops chamomile oil
- 1 ounce St. John's wort oil

Combine ingredients. Apply externally directly over problem area one or two times a day.

WARTS

Warts are raised areas on the skin that are often bumpy and dark in color. Genital warts are caused by the human papilloma virus (HPV). Difficult to detect, genital warts will temporarily turn whitish if you dab on vinegar that has been diluted in an equal amount of water.

Tea tree and particularly thuja essential oils are two of the most effective wart removers. Thuja is very strong, so use it carefully. Essential oils often get rid of warts, although the virus does stay in the system and can pop out again. For some reason, the aromatherapy treatment works in some cases, but not in others.

WART OIL 1

- 12 drops tea tree oil
- 12 drops thuja oil
- 1 teaspoon castor oil (or a carrier oil)
- 800 IU vitamin E oil

Combine the ingredients. Apply directly to the wart(s) two to four times daily. Castor oil is a good choice of oil since it is a folk treatment for warts. Adding vitamin E facilitates healing. It can be obtained by pricking two 400 IU capsules with a pin and squeezing out the contents. This is a high concentration of essential oil, and thuja is particularly strong, so use a glass rod applicator, dropper, or cotton swab to apply and be sure not to get it on the skin around the wart since repeated use can burn sensitive skin.

WART OIL 2

- 9 drops cypress oil
- 8 drops lavender oil
- 8 drops lemon oil
- 2 drops myrrh oil

Combine the ingredients. Apply as recommended with Wart Oil 1, using a glass rod applicator, dropper, or cotton swab, and take the same precautions.

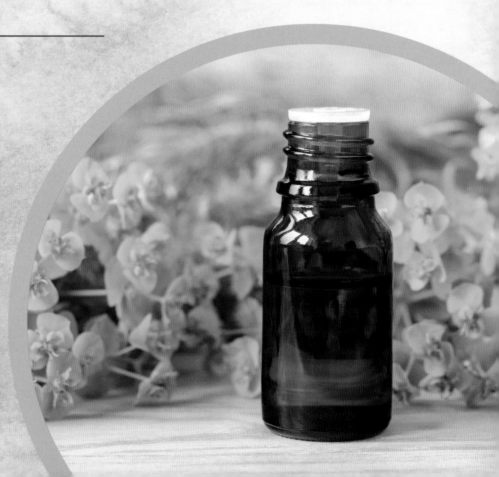

WRINKLES

Skin loses its elasticity as we age, causing wrinkles to form. Essential oils cannot magically remove wrinkles, but they can support skin elasticity, promote healthy skin, and mitigate some of the effects of aging. If you already have a good skin cream, consider simply adding in a few drops of lavender oil. Lavender soothes tired-looking skin and is a powerful free radical scavenger. Rose oil is a fantastic anti-aging resource for your blends as well. It is particularly effective for dry aging skin. However, rose oil is extremely expensive.

CARROT-GERANIUM REJUVENATING SPRAY

* 24 drops carrot seed oil
* 24 drops geranium oil
* 4 ounces water

Combine the ingredients and store in a dark glass bottle fitted with a spray top. Shake well before using. Spray on face and neck before moisturizing.

LIFTING AND SMOOTHING BLEND

* 4 drop carrot seed oil
* 4 drops rose oil
* 4 drops sandalwood oil
* 1 ounce apricot kernel, evening primrose, or grapeseed carrier oil.

Combine all ingredients and store in a dark glass bottle. Shake well before using. Apply a few drops in problems areas and rub in gently.

ANTI-AGING SERUM

* 8 drops cypress oil
* 8 drops geranium oil
* 6 drops frankincense oil
* 4 drops helichrysum oil
* 3 tbsp evening primrose carrier oil
* 3 tbsp rosehip carrier oil

Combine all ingredients and store in a dark glass bottle. Shake well before using. Apply a few drops in problems areas and rub in gently.

CLEANING APPLICATIONS AND SOAPS

The sheer variety of powerful, specialized chemical cleaners that consumers have access to in the marketplace is, on one hand, an example of the spectacular accomplishments of modern chemistry. On the other hand, it offers us the vista of slowly growing environmental degradation—toxins in our soils, polluted air and drinking water, and decreasing biodiversity. The use of essential oils in place of dangerous cleaning chemicals can mitigate our toxic footprints. With a little knowledge, essential oils can be substituted for chemical cleaners. They can be used to kill bathroom mold, disinfect countertops, and repel pests and vermin. And they can do these things without leaving residual toxins that make their way into our bodies and down our drains.

There's another reason for using essential oils for housecleaning—they smell fantastic! Some people are very sensitive to the harsh and powerful fumes of commercial cleaners. They find it necessary to open windows and doors while cleaning and stay out of the rooms they've cleaned until the smells have dissipated. This is hardly the case with essential oils. In fact, cleaning with essential oils can be a pleasure. The sparkling clean scents of pine, lemon, lime, and tea tree are naturally uplifting. Lingering aromas like cedar, lavender, clary sage, and basil reinforce the feeling of a job well done.

Making your own essential-oil-based cleaning recipes doesn't take much time. It isn't expensive either. But you will want to invest in some good, dark-tinted cleaning containers and spray bottles that are made of glass. Remember that dark glass prevents the volatile compounds of the oils from losing their efficacy. And essential oils will degrade plastic containers, possibly leaching toxins from the plastic right into your cleaning solutions.

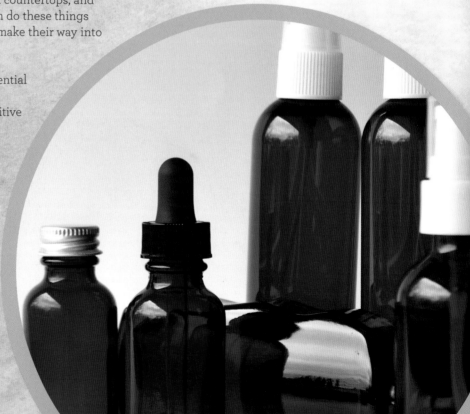

BATHROOM

The bathroom is one of the best places to use essential oils for cleaning. You'll find that tea tree and eucalyptus frequently appear in bathroom cleaning blends. They're powerful cleaners and microbe killers, they combat mold and soap residue, and they have brisk and clean aromas. But there are a number of other useful oils to consider for bathroom-specific blends, including basil, cinnamon, grapefruit, peppermint, rosemary, and thyme. And if it's cold and flu season, consider adding ravensara to your cleaning blends. Ravensara is a powerful antiviral oil.

SOAP SCUM TILE CLEANER

- 10 drops eucalyptus oil
- 10 drops tea tree oil
- 5 drops lemon oil
- 5 drops orange oil
- 1 cup white vinegar

Combine all the ingredients in a dark glass spray bottle. When ready to use, shake bottle thoroughly. Spray on scummy areas and wipe clean.

GENERAL PURPOSE BATHROOM CLEANER

- 30 drops tea tree oil
- 20 drops orange oil
- 2 cups distilled water
- 2 tbsp castile soap
- 1 tbsp baking soda

Combine all ingredients in a dark glass spray bottle. When ready to use, shake bottle thoroughly and spray on problem areas. This cleaner can be used to clean or wipe up spills and residue in tubs, tiles, floors, and sinks.

BATHROOM AIR FRESHENER

- 10 drops cilantro oil
- 10 drops rosemary oil
- 5 drops lemon oil
- 5 drops lemongrass oil
- 5 drops lime oil
- 5 drops litsea cubeba oil
- 1 tbsp rubbing alcohol
- 1/2 cup distilled water

Combine all ingredients in a dark glass spray bottle. Spray in the air when the room needs to be freshened.

TOILET BOWL CLEANER

- 5 drops hyssop oil
- 5 drops pine oil
- 5 drops spruce oil
- 3 drops lemon oil
- 3 drops grapefruit oil
- 1 cup borax
- 1 cup white vinegar

Thoroughly stir the oils into the borax and store in a dark, airtight container. When ready to use, sprinkle several spoonfuls into toilet. Add vinegar and scrub. If possible, let mixture set in bowl overnight before scrubbing.

KITCHEN

DISH SOAP

- 15 drops lemon oil
- 5 drops bergamot oil
- 3 drops lavender oil
- 3 drops lime oil
- 22 ounces castile soap

Combine all ingredients in a dark glass container. Shake container gently before use.

KITCHEN COUNTER DISINFECTANT AND CLEANER

- 5 drops cypress oil
- 5 drops grapefruit oil
- 5 drops palmarosa oil
- 5 drops rosemary oil
- 5 drops tea tree oil
- 1 cup distilled water
- 1 cup vinegar

Combine all ingredients in a dark glass container. Shake container before use. Spray on problem areas and wipe clean. (Do not use this or any vinegar-based cleaning blend on granite countertops.)

SIMPLE OVEN CLEANER

- 15 drops orange oil
- 15 drops pine oil
- 10 drops tea tree oil
- 3/4 cup baking soda
- 4 tbsp water

Combine all ingredients into a paste. Apply paste over the oven area. Let it sit for 5-10 minutes. Wipe off paste and then wipe again with a wet sponge.

LINOLEUM FLOOR RESCUE

- 3 drops clove oil
- 3 drops eucalyptus oil
- 3 drops lavender oil
- 3 drops lemon oil
- 3 drops pine oil
- 1 tbsp castile soap
- 1 cup white vinegar
- 1 bucket hot water

Add all ingredients to a bucket of hot water and mop floor as usual.

If you've ever kept bananas around until they've gone bad or left orange peels in the kitchen trash can too long you've met fruit flies. These pests can be tenacious. Try diffusing any of the following in your kitchen: basil, camphor, cedarwood, cypress, hinoki, rosewood, or tea tree. Studies have shown that hinoki is an especially effective repellent. You can also make a water-diluted blend from any or all of these oils and spray them directly at the flies, around the trash can, or anywhere else they might gather.

GENERAL HOUSEHOLD

CARPET SPOT REMOVER

- 3 drops lemon oil
- 2 tbsp baking soda
- 1 tbsp white vinegar

Mix ingredients into a paste. Using a rag or sponge, work the paste into the area of the spot. Allow the paste to dry (about 20 minutes), and then vacuum the paste up. If the spot isn't completely gone, the process can be repeated.

GENERAL PURPOSE GERM-KILLING SPRAY

- 15 drops ravensara oil
- 10 drops cinnamon oil
- 5 drops clove oil
- 5 drops eucalyptus oil
- 5 drops rosemary oil
- 5 drops thyme oil
- 1 3/4 ounces distilled water
- 1 tbsp rubbing alcohol

Combine all ingredients in a dark glass spray bottle. Shake and spray in the air whenever you think germs are about.

HARDWOOD FLOOR CLEANER

- 10 drops cedarwood oil
- 5 drops peppermint oil
- 5 drops rosemary oil
- 1 1/2 cups white vinegar
- 1 1/2 cups water

Combine all ingredients in a dark glass spray bottle. Shake and spray on problem/dirty areas and wipe.

WINDOW CLEANING BLEND

- 4 drops lemongrass oil
- 4 drops palo santo oil
- 1/3 cup white vinegar
- 2/3 cup distilled water

Combine all ingredients in a dark glass spray bottle. Shake and spray on windows and clean as you usually would.

EXTRA STRONG MOLD FIGHTING SPRAY

- 5 drops cinnamon oil
- 5 drops clove oil
- 5 drops rosemary oil
- 5 drops tea tree oil
- 1 ounce distilled water
- 1 ounce rubbing alcohol

Combine all ingredients in a dark glass spray bottle. Shake and spray on problem mold patches. Allow to sit for a minute or more before wiping clean. Repeat if necessary.

FINISH AND FRESHEN LAUNDRY ZEST

- 5 drops grapefruit oil
- 4 drops lavender oil
- 3 drops lemon oil

Add oils to a small damp washcloth. Place in the dryer with sheets and bedding for a delightfully fresh and clean smell.

STEALTH BATHROOM DEODORIZER

Place 5-10 drops of the oil(s) of your choice on the inside of a toilet paper roll's cardboard tube. The aroma will disperse every time the roll is turned!

FESTIVE FIREPLACE

Add 5 or more drops of frankincense, myrrh, sage, thyme, or winter savory to a dry log and allow the oil to seep in (at least 15 minutes). Add the log to a lit fire.

PATIO FURNITURE FRESHENER

In an 8 oz. spray bottle combine 25 drops of pine oil, 20 drops of juniper oil, 15 drops of lemon oil, and 2 tbsp white vinegar. Add water to fill bottle and shake well. Spray furniture and wipe down.

SNEAKER STINK AWAY

In a small bowl, combine one half cup of baking soda with 5 drops of lavender oil, 5 drops of tea tree oil, 2 drops of peppermint oil, and 1 drop of thyme oil. Mix well and sprinkle in the offending shoes. Leave mixture in shoes overnight before discarding.

MOUSE BOUNDARY BLEND

Eucalyptus oil
Lemon oil
Peppermint oil
Cotton balls

Add a few drops of each oil (don't skimp on the peppermint) to each cotton ball. Place cotton balls in front of any suspected area where mice might be entering. (Note that although this remedy does deter rodents, it will not totally stop them.)

ANTS NOT WELCOME SPRAY

In an 8 oz. spray bottle combine 15 drops cedarwood oil, 10 drops patchouli oil, 10 drops peppermint oil, 10 drops tea tree oil, 10 drops vetiver oil, and one quarter cup of rubbing alcohol or vodka. Top off with water and shake well. Spray mixture in problem areas and entry points. Other ant-deterring oils include cinnamon, clove, lemon, lemongrass, and orange.

MUSTY UPHOLSTERY MAKEOVER

In a small bowl, combine one half cup of baking soda with 3 drops each of geranium, lavender, peppermint, and ylang ylang. Combine thoroughly and sprinkle over musty upholstery. Allow to stand at least 15 minutes, then vacuum off.

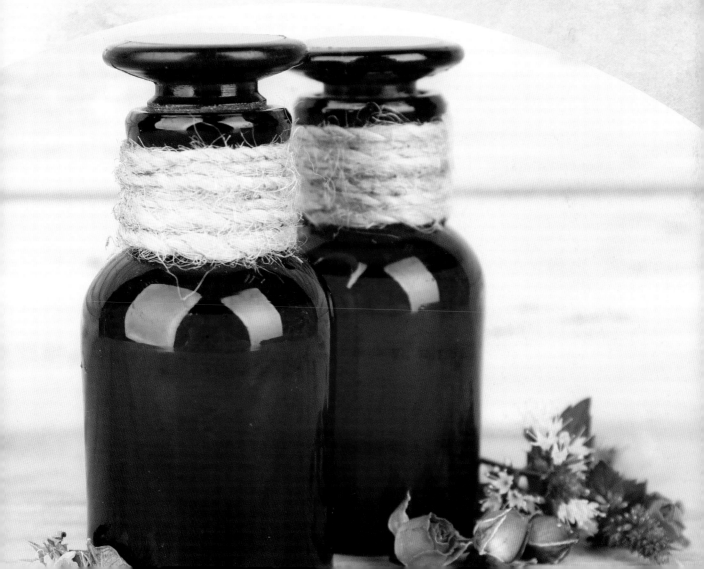

SOAPS

LAVENDER-SCENTED LIQUID SOAP

- 1 cup liquid bubble bath base
- 3/4 cup distilled water
- 1/4 teaspoon lavender oil
- 8-10 drops purple soap coloring

Combine bubble bath base, distilled water, essential oil, and coloring in a 2-cup measuring cup. Stir well. Insert funnel into a 16-ounce clear bottle with a tight-fitting cap. Pour in mixture.

LAVENDER SOAP

- 1 bar unscented white soap
- 15 drops lavender essential oil
- 5 drops rose essential oil
- 8-10 drops violet or purple soap coloring
- 1/4 cup hot distilled water
- 1/4 cup dried lavender buds or blossoms

Grate soap into medium bowl with a cheese grater. Add essential oils and soap coloring. Add the hot water and stir vigorously to distribute color evenly. Mixture will be the consistency of wet dough. Working quickly, knead in the lavender buds before the soap firms up. Form soap into 3 small balls or oval bars. Set aside on plastic wrap to dry at room temperature 24 hours.

ORANGE BLOSSOM LIQUID SOAP

- Grated peel of 1 lemon
- Grated peel of 1 orange
- 1 cup liquid bubble bath base
- 1/4 teaspoon orange blossom (neroli) oil

Combine lemon peel, orange peel and 1 cup water in small saucepan. Simmer 5 minutes. Remove from heat. Set aside to steep 1 hour. Insert funnel into a 16-ounce clear bottle with a tight-fitting cap. Place a small coffee filter in funnel. Pour lemon/orange mixture into bottle. Discard the filter and add the bubble bath base and essential oil. Seal bottle tightly and shake well.

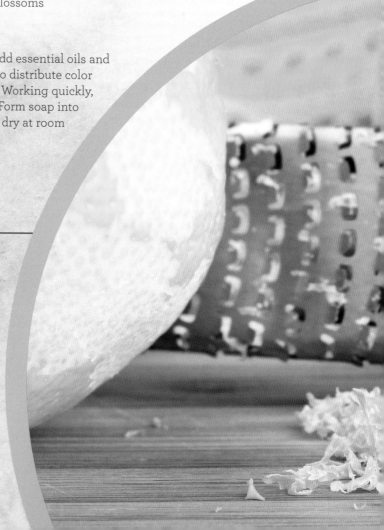

ALMOND AND TANGERINE GLYCERIN FACIAL SOAP

- 12 ounces clear or white glycerin soap base
- 1/2 cup ground raw almonds
- 1 tablespoon honey
- 15 drops tangerine or orange oil
- Sunflower oil

Lightly grease 6 muffin cups with sunflower oil. Set aside. Slice soap base into slivers. Place in microwave-safe bowl. Cover loosely with plastic wrap. Microwave on high in 20-second intervals, stirring the soap in between intervals, until the soap is liquid. Stir in almonds, honey, and tangerine oil.

Quickly pour mixture into muffin cups, filling about 3/4 full. Set aside to firm up, about 1 hour. Run a small knife around the inside edge of the muffin cups to release soap.

LEMONGRASS SOAP

- 1/2 gallon cardboard milk or orange juice carton, empty, rinsed, and dried
- 1/2 pound white vegetable soap compound
- 2 teaspoons finely minced dried or fresh lemongrass stalk
- 2-3 drops lemongrass oil

Measure 2 inches up from bottom of milk carton. Using serrated knife or scissors, cut off bottom of carton and reserve. Break or cut soap compound into 1-inch cubes. Place into 1-quart microwave safe glass measuring cup. Microwave on high in 20-second intervals or less, stirring the soap in between intervals, until the compound melts. Remove from microwave and stir in the lemongrass and essential oil (stir gently to avoid creating bubbles).

Pour the mixture into the carton and let cool 10-15 minutes. Use a toothpick or bamboo skewer to distribute lemongrass in compound, if needed. Place mold in refrigerator for 1 hour. Turn the soap out and cut into cubes.

PINK HIMALAYAN SALT GRAPEFRUIT SOAP

- 1 pound goat's milk soap base
- 1/4 cup ground pink Himalayan salt
- 10-15 drops of grapefruit oil
- Soap molds
- Coconut oil

Prepare the soap molds by lightly greasing with coconut oil. Cut soap base into chunks, and then melt in a double boiler. (The soap base can also be melted in the microwave: place chunks in a glass bowl, and microwave for 30 seconds. Stir, then microwave for 10 to 20 more seconds, until the base has melted completely.) Remove from heat and add grapefruit essential oil. Stir in salt, and pour mixture into molds. Allow soap to set for at least two hours before removing from molds.

A perfect soap to use in your morning shower, this pink Himalayan salt grapefruit soap has the familiar, citrusy scent of grapefruit to wake up your mind and uplift your mood. Pink Himalayan salt is said to detoxify the skin and balance pH, while also acting as an exfoliator. Your skin will be smooth and clean, and your shower will smell delicious!

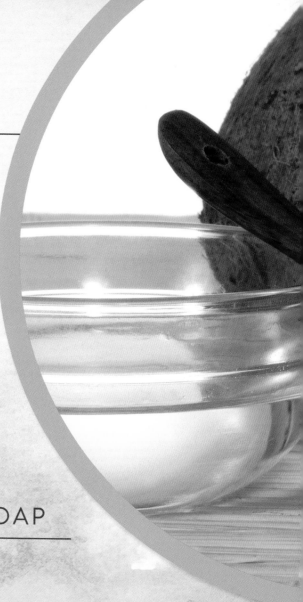

TEA TREE OIL ANTISEPTIC SOAP

- 2 cups clear glycerin soap base
- 2 tbsp tea tree oil
- Soap molds
- Coconut oil

Prepare the soap molds by lightly greasing with coconut oil. Cut glycerin soap base into chunks, and then melt in a double boiler or in the microwave (heating for 20-second intervals and stirring the soap in between intervals). Remove from heat, and stir in tea tree oil. Pour into molds, and allow to set for at least two hours.

Tea tree oil is well renowned for its antibacterial, antifungal, and antiviral properties, making this easy, do-it-yourself soap a must-have for cold and flu season. It's also excellent to have on hand to wash cuts and scrapes and protect against infection, and to soothe eczema, psoriasis, and other skin conditions. The scent is a bit medicinal, but inhaling the aroma of tea tree has also been shown to ease coughs and congestion. With all of its healthy benefits, this is a useful soap to keep in your medicine cabinet!

ELEMI AND LEMON FOAMING HAND SOAP

- 1 cup distilled water
- 4 drops of elemi oil
- 4 drops of lemon oil
- 1 tbsp unscented Castile soap
- Refillable foaming hand soap dispenser

Add distilled water and essential oils to the foaming hand soap dispenser, then add the Castile soap. Screw on the top of the dispenser and swirl to combine.

Next time you run out of store-bought foaming hand soap, don't run to the grocery store to buy more: save the empty bottle and make your own homemade version! Elemi and lemon essential oils come together to create a bright, uplifting scent, perfect for a morning aromatherapy wake-up. This is also a great soap to keep on hand in the kitchen. Elemi and lemon are both known for their antiseptic properties, so this soap will keep your hands clean while you're preparing food. And who wants fingers that smell like garlic and onions? The oils in this soap help deodorize, leaving behind a sunshiny scent!

FESTIVE EXFOLIATING SOAP

- 6 ounces shea butter soap base
- 2 tsp oats
- 7 drops cinnamon oil
- 7 drops mandarin oil
- Soap molds
- Coconut oil

Prepare the soap molds by lightly greasing with coconut oil. Cut shea butter soap base into chunks, and then melt in a double boiler or in the microwave (heating for 20-second intervals and stirring the soap in between intervals). Remove from heat, add oats and essential oils, and stir. Pour into molds, and allow to set for at least two hours.

The spicy scent of cinnamon and the sweet aroma of mandarin have long been associated with the holidays. This warm and brightly scented soap can make you feel festive any time of year! Cinnamon essential oil increases circulation and decreases inflammation in the skin, while mandarin has a calming, uplifting scent that has been shown to reduce anxiety and even nausea. And both oils help diminish skin conditions like acne and rashes. Last but not least, this soap receives some extra oomph from the addition of oats, providing gentle exfoliation.

YLANG YLANG AND BERGAMOT EXFOLIATING SOAP

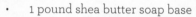

- 1 pound shea butter soap base
- 15 drops ylang ylang oil
- 10 drops bergamot oil
- 2 tbsp poppy seeds
- Soap molds
- Coconut oil

Prepare soap molds by greasing with coconut oil. Cut soap base into chunks, and melt in a double boiler or in the microwave (heating for 20-second intervals and stirring the soap in between intervals). Remove from heat, and stir in essential oils. Allow the mixture to cool slightly before stirring in the poppy seeds—this will ensure that they are evenly distributed throughout the soap, and don't sink to the bottom. Pour mixture into molds, and allow to set for at least two hours.

As the primary scent used in the famous perfume Chanel No. 5, ylang ylang has long been prized for its rich, floral scent. When it's combined with the citrusy smell of bergamot, it's perfect for creating this lovely bath soap. Not only does it smell good, but it has good-for-you benefits, as well. Ylang ylang helps prevent the signs of aging in skin, while bergamot's antiseptic properties help it fight acne and skin conditions. Poppy seeds provide natural, gentle exfoliation.

LEMON ROSEMARY GLYCERIN SOAP

- 1 pound clear glycerin soap base
- 15 drops lemon oil
- 15 drops rosemary oil
- Dried lemon peel
- Dried rosemary
- Soap molds
- Coconut oil

Prepare soap molds by greasing with coconut oil. Cut soap base into chunks, and melt in a double boiler or in the microwave (heating for 20-second intervals and stirring the soap in between intervals). Remove from heat and stir in essential oils. Place lemon peel and rosemary into soap molds, and then fill molds with soap mixture. Allow soap to set for at least two hours. Because this soap contains dried fruit and herbs, use it in a few months to prevent mold.

These soaps are as pretty as they are useful! The clear glycerin provides a versatile base for adding your own fruits and herbs. Experiment with your favorite essential oils and add-ins—try dried flower petals, tea leaves, eucalyptus, or juniper berries. This soap makes a great gift, too!

MOROCCAN SPICED HONEY SOAP

- 1 pound honey soap base
- 6 drops allspice oil
- 6 drops cardamom oil
- 6 drops cinnamon oil
- 6 drops clove essential oil
- Dried bay leaves
- Soap molds
- Coconut oil

Grease soap molds with coconut oil. Cut soap base into chunks, and melt in a double boiler or in the microwave (heating for 20-second intervals and stirring the soap in between intervals). Remove from heat and mix in all essential oils. Place a bay leaf in each mold, and fill with mixture. Allow to set for two hours before removing from molds.

With its bay leaf accent, this soap is pretty enough to place in a guest bathroom. Allspice, cardamom, cinnamon, and clove essential oils team up to provide a spicy scent and plenty of antiseptic and antioxidant benefits. Look for a melt and pour soap base with honey, which is a natural humectant and helps skin retain moisture.

TRAVEL-SIZE REFRESHING BODY WASH

- 3 1/2 tbsp unscented shower gel base
- 2 drops peppermint oil
- 1 drop rosemary oil
- 1/2 tsp jojoba oil
- 1/2 tsp vitamin E oil
- 2 ounce bottle

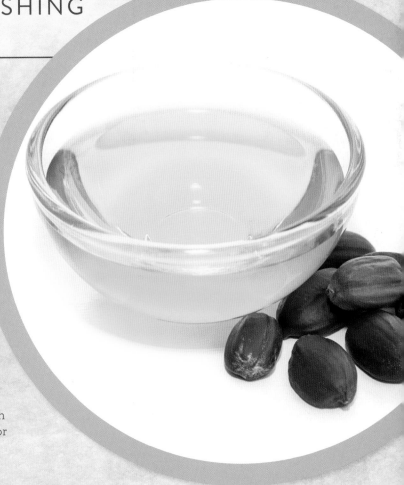

Place all ingredients into bottle, and swirl to combine. That's it!

This TSA-approved travel-size body wash will help you perk up after a long day of travel. Peppermint essential oil boosts energy and sharpens focus, while rosemary relieves stress and soothes the skin. The addition of skin-loving jojoba oil and vitamin E helps moisturize and nourish with antioxidants. This body wash doesn't lather as much as a store-bought brand, but most commercial soaps add harsh chemicals to create lather. Remember that lather does not necessarily equal clean. So enjoy this body wash without worrying about synthetic ingredients, or about getting stopped at airport security!

CUSTOMIZABLE MELT AND POUR SOAP

- 1/4 cup water
- 1/4 cup dried and crushed herbs (try lavender, lemon balm, or mint)
- 6 drops of essential oil (your choice)
- 2 cups of shredded Ivory soap
- Soap molds (optional)

Place shredded Ivory soap in a mixing bowl. In a small pan, add water, herbs, and essential oil and bring to a boil, stirring frequently. Pour the mixture over the Ivory soap and mix well, then let the soap stand for 20 minutes. When it is cool enough, divide the mixture into balls, or press into a soap mold. Once the soap has set, remove from molds, place on a glass plate or pan, and allow to dry in a cool area for at least 24 hours.

If you don't have a melt and pour soap base, this versatile recipe lets you use the soap you probably already have in your home! You can use a cheese grater or even a food processor to shred your soap bars, and then use your imagination for your herb and oil additions. Need a soap bar for a relaxing bath? Try dried lavender with chamomile essential oil. Looking for a gentle antiseptic soap to help with acne, eczema, or dermatitis? Dried rosemary with rosemary essential oil might work for you. Mix and match until you find your perfect soap!

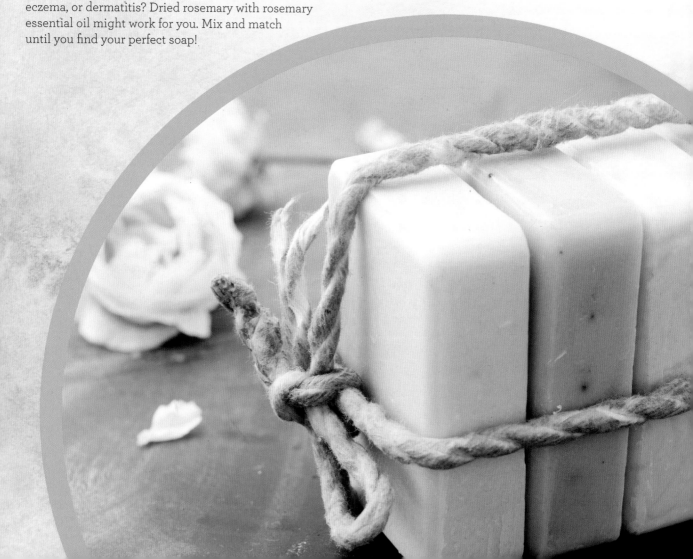